OECD DOCUMENTS

Food Safety Evaluation

PUBLISHER'S NOTE
The following texts are published in their original form to permit faster distribution at a lower cost.
The views expressed are those of the authors,
and do not necessarily reflect those of the Organisation or of its Member countries.

ORGANISATION FOR ECONOMIC CO-OPERATION AND DEVELOPMENT

ORGANISATION FOR ECONOMIC CO-OPERATION AND DEVELOPMENT

Pursuant to Article 1 of the Convention signed in Paris on 14th December 1960, and which came into force on 30th September 1961, the Organisation for Economic Co-operation and Development (OECD) shall promote policies designed:

- to achieve the highest sustainable economic growth and employment and a rising standard of living in Member countries, while maintaining financial stability, and thus to contribute to the development of the world economy;
- to contribute to sound economic expansion in Member as well as non-member countries in the process of economic development; and
- to contribute to the expansion of world trade on a multilateral, non-discriminatory basis in accordance with international obligations.

The original Member countries of the OECD are Austria, Belgium, Canada, Denmark, France, Germany, Greece, Iceland, Ireland, Italy, Luxembourg, the Netherlands, Norway, Portugal, Spain, Sweden, Switzerland, Turkey, the United Kingdom and the United States. The following countries became Members subsequently through accession at the dates indicated hereafter: Japan (28th April 1964), Finland (28th January 1969), Australia (7th June 1971), New Zealand (29th May 1973), Mexico (18th May 1994) and the Czech Republic (21st December 1995). The Commission of the European Communities takes part in the work of the OECD (Article 13 of the OECD Convention).

© OECD 1996
Applications for permission to reproduce or translate all or part of this
publication should be made to:
Head of Publications Service, OECD
2, rue André-Pascal, 75775 PARIS CEDEX 16, France.

Foreword

In *Safety Evaluation of Foods Derived through Modern Biotechnology – Concepts and Principles* (published by the OECD in 1993) it was demonstrated that the most practical approach to establishing the safety of a new food is to determine whether it is substantially equivalent to analogous conventional foods. Following up on the work that went into the preparation of that publication, the OECD Workshop on Food Safety Evaluation, held in Oxford, England, on 12-15 September 1994, looked at strategies which could be used to establish food safety **when no conventional counterpart exists for comparison**.

The value of sharing experience with novel foods from non-biotechnological sources, as well as experience with biotechologically based foods as compared with conventional counterparts, was recognized. The papers presented at the Oxford Workshop, and published here, therefore contain information on a number of aspects of the safety evaluation of novel foods. These Workshop presentations were followed by two Working Group sessions, during which strategies for establishing the safety of new foods were examined. A report of the Working Group discussions is included here.

This publication was prepared by the OECD Environment Directorate, in collaboration with the Directorate for Science, Technology and Industry. The Committee for Scientific and Technological Policy recommended derestriction. *Food Safety Evaluation* is being published on the responsibility of the Secretary-General of the OECD.

Table of Contents

Opening Remarks: The Background and Objectives of the Workshop
David Jonas, Workshop Chairman, *United Kingdom* 7

Lessons Learned from the Toxicological Testing of Irradiated Foods
David Hattan, Keynote Speaker, *United States* 11

Presentations

Construction of Safe Recombinant Wine Yeast Strains
D. Ramón, J.A. Pérez-González, L. González-Candelas, R. González,
S. Vallés, F. Piñaga, A. Querol, P. Sánchez, M.V. Gallego,
M.D. Calvo and J.E. Pérez-Ortín, *Spain* 25

Safety Approaches to Pure Culture Fermentation of Vegetables
Antonio de Castro, *Spain* 31

Demonstration of Safety: Myco-protein
P.J. Rodgers, *United Kingdom* 39

Food Safety Assessment of Transgenic Insect-resistant Bt Tomatoes
H.A. Kuiper and H.P.J.M. Noteborn, *the Netherlands* 50

Evaluation of Toxicological Studies on Flavr Savr Tomato
David Hattan, *United States* 58

Safety Evaluation of Glyphosate-tolerant Soybeans
Roy L. Fuchs, Diane B. Re, Steve G. Rogers, Bruce G. Hammond
and Stephen R. Padgette, *United States* 61

Food Safety Evaluation of a Transgenic Squash
Hector Quemada, *United States* 71

**Evaluation of Strategies for Food Safety Assessment of Genetically
Modified Agricultural Products – Information Needs**
E.J. Kok and H.A. Kuiper, *the Netherlands* 80

Limitations of Whole Food Feeding Studies in Food Safety Assessment
Bruce Hammond, Steve G. Rodgers and Roy L. Fuchs, *United States* 85

(continued on next page)

The Concept of Substantial Equivalence: Toxicological Testing of Novel Foods
Norman R. Lazarus, *United Kingdom* 98

Dietary Assessment Related to the Safety Evaluation of Foods
Michael Nelson, *United Kingdom* 107

The Role of Databases: The Example of a Food Plant Database
J. Gry, I. Søborg and I. Knudsen, *Denmark* 118

The Use of *in vivo* and *in vitro* Models in the Testing of Microorganisms
Bodil Lund Jacobsen, *Denmark* 130

The Application of Human-type Diets in Rodent Feeding Studies for the Safety Evaluation of Novel Foods
A.C. Huggett, M. Marchesini, I. Perrin, B. Schilter, J.C. Tschantz, A. Donnet, P. Morgenthaler, G. Sunahara and H-P. Würzner, *Switzerland* 135

Investigations of the Allergenicity of Brazil Nut 2S Seed Storage Protein in Transgenic Soybean
J.A. Nordlee, S.L. Taylor, J.A. Townsend, L.A. Thomas and R. Townsend, *United States* 151

US EPA Considerations for Mammalian Health Effects Presented by Transgenic Plant Pesticides
John L. Kough, *United States* 156

Annex I: Report of the Working Group Sessions 163

Annex II: List of Participants 169

OECD Environmental Health and Safety Publications 175

Opening Remarks:
The Background and Objectives of the Workshop

David Jonas (Workshop Chairman)

**Ministry of Agriculture, Fisheries and Food
United Kingdom**

Introductory remarks

I should first like to welcome you all to Oxford and to this Workshop on food safety sponsored by the OECD. I can see that I have many old friends in the room, but for those of you who do not know me I am David Jonas and I work with the Food Science Group of the Ministry of Agriculture, Fisheries and Food (MAFF) here in the UK. We have more than 60 delegates here from some 20 OECD countries and international organisations. Delegates are present from governments, from industry, and from the academic community. I am particularly pleased that we have delegates from Mexico, which only became a full member of the OECD a few weeks ago.

I should like to say a few words about the background to this Workshop and how it fits into a number of initiatives in the area of food safety.

Background to the Workshop

Firstly, I should emphasize that this is an OECD-sponsored Workshop and that we in the UK Ministry of Agriculture, Fisheries and Food are pleased to have the opportunity to host it here in Oxford. The Workshop also enjoys the collaborative support of the World Health Organization. In addition to my role as chairman of the technical session, I am here representing that organisation.

The OECD came into being in 1961. Its remit is, essentially, to promote policies which are designed to further growth and employment in Member countries and which contribute to world economic development and world trade. In 1983, the OECD Committee for Science and Technology established a Group of National Experts (GNE) on Safety in Biotechnology. This group developed many publications which have been instrumental in informing and shaping the policies of Member countries towards the safety of biotechnology.

In 1990 the GNE agreed that work on food safety, with particular attention given to the elaboration of scientific principles for assessing the safety of new foods or food components produced by means of biotechnology, was of high priority and should be initiated as soon as possible. The GNE established a working group on food safety to take the matter forward and Frank Young of the United States was elected Chairman. Under his dynamic chairmanship, the working group developed *Safety Evaluation of Foods Derived by Modern Biotechnology – Concepts and Principles*, published by the OECD in 1993. The main thrust of this report was that the most practical approach to the determination of the safety of a new food is to consider whether the new food is substantially equivalent to analogous conventional foods, if such exist.

The report left two questions unanswered. Firstly, it covered only foods of terrestrial origin; and secondly, it covered only those foods which had acceptable counterparts with which they could be compared.

The first question was addressed at an OECD symposium on Aquatic Biotechnology and Food Safety which took place in Bergen, Norway, in June 1992. The report of that symposium was published by the OECD in 1994 as *Aquatic Biotechnology and Food Safety*. Essentially, it was concluded at the symposium that, with certain caveats, the principles established for the products of terrestrial biotechnology also applied to aquatic biotechnology.

This Workshop here in Oxford was established primarily to address the second question, i.e. what strategies can be used to establish the safety of food produced by biotechnology if there is no acceptable counterpart for comparison. In planning the Workshop, the Food Safety Working Group recognized that biotechnology-derived products were not unique in respect of their safety assessment. We would need to look more generally at food safety assessment. In developing a strategy for the assessment of biotechnology-based products without conventional counterparts, we would need to learn from experiences with novel foods from non-biotechnological sources, as well as from experiences with biotechnology-based foods with conventional counterparts. What would emerge could form the basis of approaches to the safety assessment of any foods without conventional counterparts.

Our task, as set out for us by the Food Safety Working Group, is to review current knowledge and experience with respect to methods for the safety evaluation of new foods. Over the next three days, therefore, we will evaluate experiences gained through specific case studies, review existing and new methodologies for food safety evaluation, and consider testing strategies and principles for the safety assessment of foods. In doing so, we will need to bear in mind the definition of safe use which the OECD has established. With respect to food and food components, safe use is that which presents a socially acceptable risk under expected conditions of consumption.

As many of you will know, the Group of National Experts on Safety in Biotechnology no longer exists as such although its work continues. With its demise, its various working groups also ceased to exist although ongoing activities such as this Workshop have proceeded. The output from this Workshop will nevertheless be of value to the OECD and its Member countries, and I am assured that the report will be made available in the usual way.

I see this Workshop as being part of a much wider international activity in relation to biotechnology and food safety. It is therefore appropriate to say a few words about what is going on internationally in relation to biotechnology and food safety, and how this Workshop fits in with these activities.

Many individual countries have developed or are developing procedures for assessing the safety of foods produced by biotechnology for application within their own borders. These countries include Canada, Japan, the Netherlands, the Nordic countries, the UK and the US. There are doubtless others. Although these various strategies have much in common, there are also differences. It is these differences that have the potential to lead to barriers to trade in foods produced using biotechnology.

There is no doubt that biotechnology can have a major role to play in meeting future world demands for food. This Workshop provides us with the opportunity to provide the scientific foundations for an internationally harmonized approach to the safety evaluation of new foods and particularly new biotechnology-derived foods.

Perhaps the first attempts at international guidelines on assessing the safety of foods were those developed in the late 1970s and early 1980s by the Protein Advisory Group of the United Nations – later to become part of the United Nations University. These guidelines, of course, predate the development of genetic modification and the modern techniques of biotechnology.

Over the following years biotechnology advanced enormously, and in 1990 the World Health Organization and the UN's Food and Agriculture Organization organized an expert consultation which developed a strategic approach to the assessment of foods produced by biotechnology. This was published in 1991. The WHO sponsored a Workshop to examine the health aspects of marker genes in genetically modified plants in 1993. The Workshop report is available from WHO. That Workshop, held in Copenhagen, would not have taken place without the generous support of the Nordic Council. WHO is grateful that the Nordic Council has also agreed to support a further Workshop in Copenhagen later this year with a view to examining the practical application of substantial equivalence principles.

The Codex Alimentarius Commission was established in 1962 to implement the joint food standards programme of FAO and WHO. The Commission has indicated its intention of developing Codex Guidelines for the safety assessment of foods produced by biotechnology for presentation to the Commission in 1997, and also perhaps a general standard for biotechnological-based foods. Codex Guidelines and Standards have assumed a new importance in world trade following last year's GATT agreements. I see these documents as being the culmination of all of our activities over the past few years.

Hopefully, you will now be clearer as to the importance of the task before us over the next few days and its relationship to other activities.

Organisation of the Workshop

Let me now say a few words about the structure of the Workshop.

In a few minutes David Hattan from the United States will be talking about experiences with the safety testing of irradiated foods. This will be a useful introduction to our discussions, since irradiated foods were amongst the first whole foods to be subjected to systematic safety evaluation. We can learn a lot from these experiences. The fate of food irradiation and the unacceptability of irradiated foods to many consumers serves to remind us what could happen to the products of biotechnology if consumers are not convinced as to the rigour of their safety evaluation, since consideration of the fate of food irradiation shows us what could happen to foods produced using biotechnology.

We hope you will use the time after David Hattan's talk and over dinner this evening to get to know one another, so that tomorrow we can have really uninhibited discussions.

Tomorrow we start by examining a series of case studies of tests and testing strategies applied to foods and major food components. This will be followed by consideration of the present state of the art in various tests for addressing human health targets. Tomorrow's dinner is sponsored by the Ministry of Agriculture, Fisheries and Food and the Ministry's Chief Scientist (Food), Dr Howard Denner, will be present to say a few words.

We will conclude our consideration of testing methodologies on Wednesday morning, following which we propose holding a panel discussion. This is intended to focus on the value and limitations of various testing methods, and will help identify the issues that need to be addressed in more detail.

Detailed consideration of toxicological and nutritional methods, tests and strategies will take place in two parallel Working Groups throughout Wednesday afternoon.

On Thursday we will receive and discuss the reports of the two Working Groups.[1]

I should like to emphasize a few points:

- This is a Workshop, not a conference, and I hope you will all participate. The formal presentations will set the scene, but we are looking to you all to add your views and opinions.

- I hope we will not only hear of your successes but also of your failures, as there is much that we can all learn from each other's mistakes;

- A reminder that our discussions should focus on science. They should not be seen as a commentary on the regulatory status of the foods under discussion.

Finally, this Workshop would not have been possible without the enormous efforts of a number of people. I would like particularly to acknowledge in this respect Peter Kearns of the OECD, and Ranjini Rasaiah and Pendi Najran of MAFF.

---

[1] See Annex I.

Lessons Learned from the Toxicological Testing of Irradiated Foods

David Hattan, Keynote Speaker

United States Food and Drug Administration

The toxicological testing and safety assessment of irradiated foods has what one might characterize as a tortuous or at least checkered history. A portion of the problem for the US Food and Drug Administration can be traced to the insistence of the US Congress that, as a part of the food additives amendment of 1958, the process of irradiating foods be demonstrated to be as safe as food additives. Sec. 201 (s) of the Federal Food, Drug and Cosmetic Act states that

> *The term "food additive" means any substance the intended use of which results or may reasonable be expected to result, directly or indirectly, in its becoming a component or otherwise affecting the characteristics of any food (including any substance intended for use in producing, manufacturing, packing, processing, preparing, treating, packaging, transporting, or holding food; and including any source of radiation intended for any such use)....*

Both the Congress and the regulatory agencies involved were aware that food irradiation was a process and not a food additive; however, the Congress meant for this particular food processing technology to meet the same standard of safety as food additives (Pauli and Takeguchi, 1986).

No other food process has been subjected to this same rigorous safety requirement. Knowing some of the physical and chemical changes that occur in foods when they have been exposed to other preparative and preservation treatments such as canning, baking, broiling, browning, etc., it is conceivable that they too would not be readily accepted if one were to insist that they provide rigorous evidence of safety.

In 1954, officials of the US Food and Drug Administration (US FDA) published an article listing certain requirements for the toxicological testing of irradiated foods, including the need for long-term studies (Lehman and Lang, 1954). The interest in and sponsorship of long-term studies was elicited from the US government when the US Army conducted a feasibility experiment on the process of food irradiation and, based on results from organoleptic and biological tests, concluded that this process could enable the production of wholesome, good-tasting, economical and shelf-stable products for field rations. It was anticipated that the process might reduce dependence on refrigeration and greatly reduce food-handling costs for the military (Pauli and Takeguchi, 1986). Subsequently, the US government spent millions of dollars and more than a decade attempting to supply results from high-quality feeding studies that would establish the safety of the food irradiation process over a span of doses and technical uses.

Results of early studies with irradiated foods

While a great deal was ultimately learned about the potential "toxicity" of whole foods, both irradiated and non-irradiated, there were numerous setbacks along the way. In a series of articles published in the *Journal of the American Institute of Nutrition* (1960), the principal investigators of a number of studies recounted their experiences with the toxicologic testing of irradiated foods.

One of the studies (Richardson et al., 1960) reported that when rats were fed irradiated foods (green beans – 2.8 Kgy, and chicken – 5.6 Kgy) for long periods, reproductive and growth measurements were comparable. However, there was apparently a higher incidence of blindness (microphthalmia) in the groups receiving irradiated foods versus non-irradiated foods.

The comparative incidence of blindness over four generations was: F_0 = 49/856 or 5.7 per cent; F_1 = 44/732 or 6.0 per cent; F_2 = 39/587 or 6.6 per cent; and F_4 = 5/389 or 1.3 per cent. Overall, the comparative rates were: irradiated foods 5.34 per cent, and controls 1.61 per cent. The experiment was repeated twice. The successive incidence of microphthalmia was: irradiated groups 5.34, 1.6 and 1.7 per cent; and non-irradiated groups, 1.6, 0.6 and 1.7 per cent. In these three experiments, over 8500 rats were monitored for this effect.

The investigators convinced themselves ultimately that this was not a treatment-related effect by measuring the rates of blindness in 16 other experiments conducted for other purposes. These 16 studies involved numerous and diverse diet treatments. The rates of blindness varied from 0.55 to 8.6 per cent for the individual treatment groups. About 4200 rats were examined in these 16 studies. Thus, it required the examination of over 12,000 rats to finally resolve what turned out to be a fortuitous occurrence of blindness in the irradiated foods group (Richardson et al., 1960).

The results of a second study were reviewed by an experimenter at the Department of Anatomy, University of Illinois (Monsen, 1960). In this particular study, mice of the Strong A and Strong Cb strains were used as the test subjects. There was a mixture of foods: pork loin – 8.8 per cent, chicken – 6.6 per cent, milk – 19.3 per cent, white potatoes – 22.9 per cent, and carrots – 43 per cent. This mixture was dried and was added as 20 per cent of the diet. All foods except the potatoes received a radiation dose of 56 Kgy. Potatoes received about 110 Gy. A vitamin supplement was added daily to the dietary mixture.

By 19 months into this long-term study, 17.5 per cent of the test mice had died of complications to the left atrial dilation (or 70 per cent of the current mortality of the test animals). The affected atrial segment was so distended that it displaced the contents of the mouse's thorax downward and to the right. Subsequent testing was not successful in definitively specifying the basis of the lower lesion; however, when the mice were fed only evaporated milk, the "exploding heart" effect was manifested more in the irradiated, cooked milk group (85 per cent) than in the irradiated, uncooked milk (13.6 per cent incidence). The most likely cause of this effect was some type of dietary deficiency (avitaminosis?), according to the authors (Monsen, 1960).

In a third study (Johnson et al., 1960), Sprague-Dawley derived rats were used in a long-term experiment with irradiated beef (56 Kgy). Within 42 days of the onset of the study, the male rats began to die of hemorrhagic complications. Using a series of experiments with increasing levels of vitamin K supplementation, the authors were able to establish conclusively that the original diet was marginal in vitamin K content and that the irradiation of the beef intensified that deficiency state. The results of the study established that, in this strain of rats, the male requires more vitamin K in the diet than the female.

The results of studies such as those reported above suggest that the early experiments with irradiated foods provided the opportunity to study and establish the nutritional requirements of animals being subjected to an inadvertently unbalanced source of micronutrient. Thus, the investigators were required to determine what the basic requirements for nutrition were for the experimental subjects when fed *either* irradiated or non-irradiated foods.

Affirmation of testing requirements for safety assessment

In 1967, the US FDA reconsidered the toxicological testing needs for irradiated foods and developed a list of questions that needed to be answered before the process could be considered safe (Anonymous, 1967). This 1967 series of recommendations included a discussion of both the toxicologic and nutritional questions that remained to be answered for irradiated foods.

Two general questions were set forth for the nutritional component: 1) If a food is an important source of one or more nutrients or nutritional properties or qualities essential for optimum health in any diet, does the proposed irradiation treatment of the food cause it to be adulterated or devalued such that it is nutritionally inferior to the non-irradiated food? and 2) If yes, does it pose a potential public health nutrition risk for individuals in the population?

In the 1967 guidance document, nutritional quality consisted of the following:

1) vitamin content, stability, and physiological availability;

2) fat content, quality, and essential fatty acid composition;

3) protein quality;

4) digestibility of fats, proteins and carbohydrates, and availability of energy derived from them;

5) absence of antimetabolites;

6) absence of toxic degradation products of radiation-sensitive nutrients and food additives; and

7) subjective qualities of food that make it desirable to eat.

The toxicological testing requirements for establishing the safety of irradiated foods essentially re-emphasized those raised by the 1954 article by FDA officials. Acute studies were viewed as being of little or no value, because it was believed that any effects that might be observed were likely to be subtle and therefore unlikely to be detected in short-term studies (Anonymous, 1967).

Carcinogenic and reproductive effects were to be assessed with lifetime studies in two species, one rodent and the other non-rodent. The number of animals was to be 20 rodents (rats) and four non-rodents (dogs) per test group. The test groups were to include a non-irradiated control group and two irradiated; one at 1X the requested radiation dose and another at 2X (Anonymous, 1967).

The test material was to be added to the diet in quantities as high as practicable, but without introducing nutritional incompatibilities or other effects solely attributable to the food. Thirty-five per cent of the diet was the maximum level of addition of irradiated food to the test diet generally recommended, unless there was reason to believe the animals would suffer adverse effects unrelated to the test materials. The diets were to be nutritionally balanced, and the toxicological studies were not to be used to study nutritional relationships or changes induced in the food by the irradiation treatment (Anonymous, 1967).

Finally, statistical design was to be determined by consultation with a competent biostatistician, the histology reports were to provide detailed descriptions of pathology by individual tissue, and the descriptions were to be provided by a pathologist (Anonymous, 1967).

Early petitions for irradiated foods

In the 1960s the FDA promulgated several regulations for the use of irradiation of different food products: canned bacon at an irradiation dose of 45-65 Kgy for sterilization, and potatoes at a dose of 0.05 to 0.1 Kgy for sprout inhibition. The submission of a petition for irradiated ham that relied on the studies previously submitted for other products induced the FDA to ask the petitioners to provide the original data sets for the irradiated food studies. The agency concluded after evaluation of the original data that adverse effects may have been observed and not adequately reported in the previously submitted data summaries from the earlier studies, although the numbers of animals used were too small to be sure that such effects were caused by the irradiated food. The result of this re-evaluation was that the FDA revoked the approval of the sterilizing dose for canned bacon (Pauli and Takeguchi, 1986).

Agency re-examination of testing requirements

By 1980, the FDA was still unwilling to accept the toxicological testing information available at that time as being adequate to assure the safety of a number of applications of irradiation to foods. It was decided to charge another group of scientists within the FDA Bureau of Foods (now known as the Center for Food Safety and Applied Nutrition) to re-examine the previous bases for FDA recommendations for toxicological testing, and to judge whether the accumulating data in other scientific fields, such as radiation chemistry, might contribute to an understanding of the risk potential of radiation-induced changes in food and allow the FDA to modify its recommendations on the toxicologic testing required for irradiated foods. This task force was referred to as the Bureau of Foods Irradiated Food Committee (BFIFC).

In its report the task force concluded that:

1) Calculations from radiation chemistry clearly indicate that irradiation doses of 1 Kgy (or 100 krad) or less yield a concentration of total radiolytic products in food that is so limited that it would be difficult to detect and subsequently measure their potential toxicological properties. (Based on these calculations, there should be no more than 3 mg of radiolytic products per kg of irradiated food at an irradiation dose of 100 krad.)

2) Foods irradiated at 1 Kgy or less or at 50 Kgy (but constituting no more than 0.01 per cent of the diet) are safe to consume without additional toxicological testing.

3) It is recommended to have genotoxicity testing of concentrated extracts of radiolytic products extracted from irradiated foods.

4) Due to the potentially large molecular weights of some of the radiolytic products, it is recommended that they be subjected to enzymatic digestion before genotoxicity testing.

5) Foods irradiated above 1 Kgy must be evaluated in a 90-day feeding study in a rodent and a non-rodent species.

6) To enhance the level of exposure to the radiolytic products incorporated into the diet of the test species, the test materials may be subjected to lyophilization before incorporation into the diet.

7) Because the radiolytic products formed are more determined by the chemical composition of the food than by the irradiation dose, when two or more foods are of sufficient similarity with respect to chemical composition and conditions of irradiation, they may be reviewed in common for regulatory purposes.

The report and the accompanying recommendations of this Bureau of Foods task force on irradiated foods (the so-called BFIFC report) provided the conceptual basis for the FDA to regulate certain types of radiation treatment of foods (Brunetti et al., 1980).

Analysis of toxicologic studies on irradiated foods

Following the 1981 Joint FAO/IAEA/WHO report on Wholesomeness of Irradiated Foods, the FDA's Bureau of foods established another group of scientists, the Irradiated Foods Task Force (IFTG), to review all available toxicological data on irradiated foods up to that date. In the process of evaluating the data, the IFTG collected and summarized the data pertaining to irradiated foods, identified any recurring adverse findings, assessed the presence of patterns and trends among the various studies, and summarized the overall results at the end of the review (Pauli and Takegichi, 1986).

The IFTG reviewed about 400 toxicological studies. Of that 400, over 250 were "accepted" or "accepted with reservations" for review. Studies were rejected for the following reasons:

1) The dose of irradiation was not reported.

2) The dose of irradiation was less than 0.1 Kgy or more than 100 Kgy.

3) The number of animals used per group was not reported.

4) The number of rodents used was less than five per test group.

5) The diet fed was determined to be nutritionally inadequate.

6) The study was conducted without a non-irradiated control.

7) Irradiated food was administered by some means other than orally.

8) The type of food irradiated was not reported.

9) The studies were performed by the Industrial Biotest Laboratories, which was determined to be in violation of US FDA Good Laboratory Practices regulations.

It was the conclusion of the IFTG that the studies that were "accepted with reservation" could not stand alone as adequate evidence supporting the safety of the irradiated food tested; but that if several such studies (with differing design limitations) presented the same results, that is, no consistent indication of an adverse effect(s), this was collectively important information of a lack of adverse effect.

On even more detailed examination, only 69 studies were carried forward as useful for supporting the safety of irradiated foods. Among those accepted and accepted with reservation categories, additional deficiencies were discovered: 1) problems associated with diet, and 2) inadequate experimental design.

Some examples are listed below:

1) Dietary problems

    a) general dietary, vitamin, mineral and/or protein deficiency

    b) restricted food intake

    c) unpalatable diet, e.g. increased peroxidation of oils

2) Inadequate experimental design

    a) inadequate control diet

    b) "replicate" experiments

c) too few animals/sex/group, use of one sex, or numbers of animals were not reported

d) combining of data such as "total tumors" which is currently considered inappropriate

e) inadequate presentation of the final report, or insufficient data for evaluation, e.g. only a data summary was presented

f) addition of antioxidants such as BHT to diet either before or after irradiation

g) insufficient recovery time for female animals between breedings in a reproduction study

h) lack of random selection of animals for groups

i) questionable culling practices, and/or sibling matings in reproduction studies

j) inadequate histopathology

k) use of animals too old for breeding purposes

l) addition of extra animals in the middle of experiments

m) inadequate length of time for a study, e.g. carcinogenicity

The IFTG concluded that, based on their extensive review of the data, irradiated foods do appear to cause adverse effects (the overall results of these analyses may be viewed in part in Tables 1 and 2, Appendix I, of the group's report). The group did, however, express some concern over the use of traditional feeding studies to assess the potential toxicity of irradiated foods. This concern was caused by the nature of the materials tested, i.e. the extreme dilution of radiolytic products in the dietary matrix and the inability to increase the concentration of the radiolytic products in irradiated foods (US FDA Memorandum, 9 April 1982).

Actually one might make the point, in retrospect admittedly, that irradiated foods were the first "novel foods". Our insistence, based on previous experience at that time with more potent food additive materials, that we test irradiated foods at as high a level in the diet as possible led to many of the spurious and initially troubling findings of the early studies on irradiated foods. The levels of micronutrient substances, such as vitamins, were marginal in some of the diets used in the early studies. In addition, it was not always fully appreciated at the time what indeed the nutritional requirements were for the various test species. Then if one appreciates that the irradiation process itself may further reduce the concentration of certain vital nutrients, it is little wonder that the early studies produced results that were difficult, even impossible, to explain or interpret.

This characteristic of novel foods to include substances that are food-like in nature, and that imply substantial to clearly high exposures in food, produces a familiar dilemma.

How does one assure the safety of a material when the usual safety margins that toxicologists are accustomed to dealing with are no longer available because of the inherent properties of the test materials? Below I have attempted to present some of the factors that I believe one must consider in attempting to accumulate evidence for novel foods that will hopefully replace the usually comforting margin the test material enjoys between its no-observed-effect dose and the level of dietary exposure.

Identity of the macroadditive

It is important to develop a complete characterization of the source and molecular nature of each new representative of this class of food additives. The source and molecular nature of a novel food might suggest that it is so close to what occurs naturally (for which we may possess significant toxicity data) that the need for traditional toxicity testing might be meaningfully reduced. On the other hand, the source might be new and there might be little data available on the types and amounts of toxins and contaminants present. This latter situation might necessitate considerable chemical characterization and more complete toxicity testing. It may be that more resources need to be invested in exploring the nutritional effects and compatibilities than in exhaustively assessing the macroadditive's toxicological profile.

Estimated exposure levels

The estimated level of exposure to a new compound or food-like material will, of course, bear importantly on the amount and type of toxicity testing required to establish safe limits of use. For those compounds that are consumed in large quantities (multiple gram amounts), one should have excellent data on the quantities and types of impurities or contaminants. With macroadditives with this level of intake, it would be essential, for example, for the concentrations of heavy metals to be no higher than those found normally in food. If, after testing and accumulating all the information we can, we still have questions about use of the macroadditive in all possible applications, then a petition for more limited uses might be appropriate until more experience is gained with ingestion of the material. Obviously the questions remaining would have to arise only with high use, and the effect would have to be relatively minor. For example, we might want to obtain additional data on whether there are certain age groups in the general population that are more sensitive to the laxation effects of a compound.

Potential gastrointestinal effects

Some of these substances reduce caloric or fat intake by remaining largely unchanged and unabsorbed in the gastrointestinal tract. For this reason, it is quite important to know with clarity what effects may be elicited from this organ system. For example, what changes are observed in gastrointestinal function compared with those seen with more traditional foodstuffs which this macroadditive is meant to replace? Does one observe alterations in transit time of luminal contents, increased gas formation, decreased absorption of normal macronutrient portions of the diet (protein, carbohydrate and fat)? It may be necessary to perform toxicological studies with additional control groups and/or other types of special nutritional studies if there is an indication of interference with absorption or utilization of the normal macronutrients in the diet by the test material. It may be necessary, for example, to control for dietary dilution by the test substance during feeding studies. It may even be necessary to perform pilot or other kinds of special studies to separate out nutritional from toxicological effects (see below).

Testing macroadditives

A general concern that this whole class of compounds creates during toxicologic testing is the generally modest margin between the concentration tested in feeding studies and expected exposure levels to the macroadditive in foods when satisfying its intended technical function. Indeed, it is quite possible for this margin to cease to exist, i.e. for the level of exposure in foods to be virtually the same as the level tested in animal subjects.

Because of this characteristic of novel foods, it is important to carefully discern whether any effects observed in animal testing are compound-related and, if so, whether they can be expected to be manifested in humans, Even effects that might be expected and within the normal range of physiological function ordinarily, e.g. decreased transit time, might take on toxicological significance in special human populations (individuals with disorders of the lower gastrointestinal tract).

Absorption, distribution, metabolism and elimination

In like manner, to compensate for the apparent lack of dose accentuation for these substances, it would be extremely important to have excellent comparative information on the degree of absorption, distribution, metabolism and elimination. If the substance is absorbed, can the body deal effectively with the material? Is it bioaccumulated? If so, what is the organ site and does it affect organ function? What metabolites are formed? Will special toxicological studies be required to determine effects on an individual organ? What are the implications for long-term toxicological testing?

Assessment of nutritional effects

An internal FDA *ad hoc* committee created to look at the emerging issues surrounding novel foods back in the mid 1980s (Non-nutrient Foods Task Force) predicted that it would be important to have detailed information on how the substance might influence the absorption of micronutrients, such as fat and water-soluble vitamins and minerals. As our experience accumulates with these substances, it is becoming even clearer that very good data on nutritional compatibilities must be carefully collected and assessed. Thus, in comparing these materials with more traditional food additives, more time, effort and money may have to be invested in carefully characterizing the nutritional influences of these compounds. It appears logical that an expert in animal and human nutrition be added to the petitioner's research and development team at the very beginning of the development of the safety data, and that this individual should be consulted for their recommendations on nutritional questions to be considered. It is quite possible that, ultimately, this will save both time and money in the development of these macroadditives.

If one of these novel foods does adversely affect nutrition, are there ways of safely compensating for the induced nutritional changes? Do the compensatory modifications required in the formulation have other unforeseen effects that will need to be assessed? Do any of these data raise issues that will require the FDA or other regulatory entity to develop new policies regarding testing requirements, or regarding actions needed to safely use a particular macroadditive?

In addition to these questions, it may be necessary with certain macroadditives, e.g. the fat replacers, that new animal models will have to be developed and utilized to enable the macroadditive to be tested at levels that will occur with human use in foods. Commonly humans will consume 40 per cent of their calories as fat, and certain strains of rats fare poorly in long-term studies with concentrations of lipid in their diets above 10 per cent.

Need for clinical studies

In part because of the lowered dose accentuation possible with these materials, it may also be important to perform human studies with these substances. In general, it does seem appropriate that enough information be collected from current animal testing or from previous testing of the compound or very similar compounds so that any toxicities or physiological adaptations in human subjects may be anticipated. This will enable the clinical research plan to be modified to protect the participants, and to assess the compound's potential effects in the most efficient manner.

While many regulatory agencies would not approve of using human testing in lieu of animal testing for the adequate support of safety for a novel food, the final resolution of certain issues might necessitate studies on human subjects. There is precedent for this approach, as certain questions concerning the safety of a traditional food additive, aspartame, required clinical testing. In this particular case, plasma levels of phenylalllaning, glutamate and aspartate were carefully measured in human subjects following various doses of the artificial sweetener. The results of these studies assured the FDA that even high-level consumption of this artificial sweetener would not result in plasma levels of these amino acids that would place consumers at risk.

In the pursuit of information concerning how a macroadditive might affect certain human pathophysiologic states, it may be deemed appropriate for the petitioner to test whether use of the new material in certain individuals further complicates or degrades organ performance in those suffering compromised organ function.

Post-marketing surveillance

Even with the best designed protocols for human studies, incompletely answered questions may remain regarding the expected effects in human subjects. After careful consideration, the regulatory agency may recommend/agree to post-marketing surveillance as the means to supply the final increment of assurance needed for unlimited marketing of a novel food. It may be that this type of information will have to be collected from a relatively limited market area, or with greater than normal consideration for how the data are to be measured and analyzed.

Thank you all very much for your kind attention. I have attempted to review the methodological and interpretive insights that seem to me to be apparent from the experiences of testing irradiated foods. In addition, I have presented what I hope will be a useful overview of a number of factors and relationships that may be useful to consider in our attempt to assure the safety of novel foods or food-like materials.

References

Anonymous (1967) *Preparation and processing of food additive petitions: Radiation application to food.* Bureau of Science Staff Seminar, US FDA, Washington, D.C.

Anonymous (1982) *Final report of the Task Group for the review of toxicology data on irradiated foods.* US FDA Memorandum, Washington, D.C., 9 April.

Brunetti, A.P., Frattali, V., Greear, W.B., Hattan, D.G., Takeguchi, C.A. and Valcovic, L.R. (1980) *Recommendations for Evaluating the Safety of Irradiated Foods.* US Food and Drug Administration, Washington, D.C.

Johnson, B.C., Mameesh, M.S., Metta, V.C. and Rao, P.B.R. (1960) Vitamin K nutrition and irradiation sterilisation. *Fed. Proc.* 19:1038-1044.

Lehman, A.J. and Lang, E.P. (1954) Radiation sterilization V: evaluating the safety of radiation sterilized foods – FDA's official position. *Nucleonics* 12:52-54.

Monsen, H. (1960) Heart lesions in mice induced by feeding irradiated foods. *Fed. Proc.* 19:1031-1034.

Pauli, G.H. and Takeguchi, C.A. (1986) Irradiation of foods – an FDA perspective. *Fd. Rev. Internat.* 2:79-107.

Richardson, L.R., Ritchey, S.J. and Rigdon, R.H. (1960) A long-term feeding study or irradiated foods using rats as experimental animals. *Fed. Proc.* 19:1023-1027.

PRESENTATIONS

Construction of Safe Recombinant Wine Yeast Strains

D. Ramón, J.A. Pérez-González, L. González-Candelas,
R. González, S. Vallés, F. Piñaga, A. Querol, P. Sánchez,
M.V. Gallego, M.D. Calvo and J.E. Pérez-Ortín*

Departamento de Biotecnología, Instituto de Agroquímica y
Tecnología de los Alimentos, Consejo Superior de
Investigaciones Científicas, Spain

*Departamento de Bioquímica y Biología Molecular, Universidad
de Valencia, Spain

Selected dry wine yeasts

The production of wine is a complex microbiological reaction involving the sequential development of various yeast strains and lactic acid bacteria. Among these microorganisms, yeasts are primarily responsible for the alcoholic fermentation.

For many years, Spanish wines have been produced by natural fermentation caused by the sequential development of yeast populations originating from the grapes and the winery. This is the case in the Mediterranean region of Alicante. In this region, during the final stages of grape maturation, the variable climate strongly affects the composition of the microbial flora. For this reason, the quality and organoleptical characteristics of the wine vary considerably from one year to another.

In order to tackle this problem of variability, we have isolated and characterized a *Saccharomyces cerevisiae* strain (namely T73) from Alicante musts, which when used as a dry yeast produces an excellent wine.[1] This strain has been commercialized by Lallemand Inc. (Canada) and has been used at an industrial level during the last three years in different wineries of our region, solving the problem of wine quality variation.

Molecular monitoring of the population dynamics of wine fermentation

The quality of wines is a direct consequence of the evolution of the microbial flora during fermentation. Using a simple and inexpensive molecular biology method based on mtDNA restriction analysis profile,[2] we have studied the population dynamics of natural and T73 inoculated industrial wine fermentation.

Analysis of fresh must shows the presence of a great number of different wild *S. cerevisiae* strains. Curiously, only a fraction of them are present during the whole fermentation process, indicating that the must is an ecological reservoir for many different *S. cerevisiae* strains though the wine is produced by only a few of them.

In the case of natural fermentation, we observed a sequential substitution of the S. cerevisiae strains during fermentation coinciding with different fermentation phases.[3] By comparison, in inoculated fermentation the predominance of the inoculated strain is evident (60 to 90 per cent depending on the fermentation). Curiously, the inoculated S. cerevisiae does not significantly suppress the development of natural oxidative and apiculate yeast strains during the early stages of the fermentation, thus allowing their influence during this period, which could have important effects on wine flavour.[4]

From a biotechnological point of view, these results have important repercussions. Natural fermentation is a complex situation in which many different S. cerevisiae strains undergo sequential substitutions during fermentation. In the inoculated fermentation, however, a clear imposition and predominance of the inoculated dry yeast is detected. This microbiological simplification of the fermentation process opens the way to genetic modification of the active dry yeast, constructing strains which express metabolic activities that positively affect the organoleptical characteristics of the wine produced.[5]

Genetic transformation of industrial wine yeast strains

Genetic modification of an industrial yeast strain requires the development of a transformation system. Transformation of laboratory S. cerevisiae strains is now a trivial procedure. On the other hand, some of the industrial S. cerevisiae strains are recalcitrant to the uptake of exogenous DNA. This is a well-documented problem in the case of brewing yeast strains. The polyploid nature of some of the most common prototrophic markers (e.g. *leu2*, *ura3*) in industrial wine yeasts (unpublished results) makes their complementation using the cloned wild type alleles impossible. Selection of transformants therefore has to be based on dominant markers.

The T73 industrial wine yeast strain is extremely sensitive to the antibiotic cycloheximide. A selection system based on the acquisition of resistance to this antibiotic by complementation with the CYH2 gene has been developed. Transformants obtained in this way are quite stable, even in the absence of selective pressure, not only in laboratory cultures but also in microvinification experiments. In the latter case, the wines produced have exactly the same organoleptical characteristics as those produced by the industrial strain T73.[6]

From a safety point of view, the industrial use of a yeast strain expressing an antibiotic resistance gene is not desirable. In addition, the presence of bacterial DNA fragments could generate risk problems related to genetic transfer. In this respect, we are now designing reasonable alternatives (see below).

Wine aroma: a black box to manipulate

One of the most important characteristics of a quality wine is its aroma. Some authors indicate that wine's aroma is the result of the interaction of several hundred volatile compounds. The presence of monoterpenes in Muscat grapes and their role in the development of wine flavour is now well-established. These compounds are present in the must partly as free volatile forms, and partly as glycosidically bound non-volatile precursors.[7] This last fraction is a potential source of flavours which generally remain odourless in the traditional winemaking process.

Enzymatic hydrolysis of these grape glycosides has been suggested by some authors as a strategy to enhance wine flavour. Various fungal cellulases and hemicellulases have been added as exogenous enzymes, with some positive results in microvinification experiments.[8] In fact, addition of commercial enzymatic preparations is now a frequent practice in wineries.

These commercial preparations are normally obtained from fungal cultures (*Aspergillus* and *Trichoderma* species). They constitute a complex, undefined mixture of enzymes. The analysis of three of them frequently used in Spanish wineries showed the presence of multiple activities, mainly α-L-arabinofuranosidase, β-glucosidase, endo-β-(1,4)-xylanase, and polygalacturonase.[9] The composition of the mixtures is not included in the labels.

Construction of wine yeast strains expressing fungal enzymes

A previously cloned *Trichoderma longibrachiatum egl1* gene encoding a β-(1,4)-endoglucanase activity[10] has been expressed in the T73 wine yeast strain under the control of a strong constitutive yeast promoter (the actin gene promoter) and the exogenous protein secreted to the must using the fungal signal peptide. This recombinant strain produces wine in the same way as the untransformed strain, but the concentration of some volatile compounds is increased and the aroma profile is different, being more fruity.[6] From an industrial point of view, this is a desirable change and is probably due to residual β-glucosidase activity of the EGL1 protein.

Following a similar strategy, we have expressed other fungal enzymes in the T73 strain such as a *Fusarium solani* fs. *pisi* pectate lyase and an *Aspergillus niger* α-L-arabinofuranosidase (unpublished results).

Development of safety recombinant wine yeast

There are three differences between the endoglucanolytic T73 strain and the original T73 strain:

1) The recombinant strain secretes the *T. longibrachiatum* endoglucanase to the must.

2) The recombinant strain produces wine with an altered volatile compounds profile.

3) The recombinant strain has both ampicillin and cycloheximide resistance genes, as well as prokaryotic DNA sequences.

The first difference constitutes an equivalent situation to that generated by brewing companies, in which semi-purified *Trichoderma* endoglucanases with a high degree of identity to the *T. longibrachiatum* are added directly to the must. In such cases, the concentration of the fungal enzyme in the beer must is similar to that detected in the wine must.[6] It is also interesting to note that, for some of the wine enzymatic preparations, we also detect β-(1,4)-endoglucanase activity.

With respect to the profiles of aromatic compounds, the microvinification experiments clearly showed an increase in concentration of two to three times, mainly for some major volatile compounds such as 2-butanol, isoamyl acetate and isoamyl alcohol. It is possible to detect similar, or indeed higher, final concentrations of these volatiles in other commercial wines.

The final difference is the most important from a safety point of view. There is apparently no danger to anyone consuming wine produced by this recombinant strain due to the fact that the yeast contains two antibiotic resistance genes. Neither the gene itself (which is a piece of DNA) nor the encoded protein are toxic to the consumer. In any case, after entry into the digestive tract both DNA and the protein would be broken down just like all other ingested DNA and protein. The greater risk concerns the possibility of transfer of this genetic information to other bacteria, particularly some enteric pathogenic bacteria. In this sense, the existence within the transformant of bacterial plasmid DNA sequences presents an extra risk.

In order to solve this problem, we have decided to construct new T73 endoglucanolytic strains in which only the expression cassette containing the fungal gene under the control of the actin promoter is integrated into the yeast genome. In this case, neither resistance genes nor bacterial DNA fragments will be present in the recombinant strain. This approach requires the development of transformation protocols using high-velocity microprojectiles. Using this method, it is possible to transform the T73 strain and obtain a high frequency of cotransformation (unpublished results). Cotransformation with a plasmid containing the cycloheximide gene and a linear DNA fragment comprising the expression cassette flanked by yeast rDNA sequences can generate integrative transformants of multiple copies of the construction at the ribosomal repeat unit. A subsequent curing of the plasmid containing the resistance gene can be done by growing the transformant in the absence of selective pressure.

With this kind of construction, the risk of DNA transfer from the recombinant wine yeast may be expected to be the same as that from the untransformed strain. At present we do not have information about the risk of DNA transfer from wine yeasts. It is important to note that no known DNA viruses have been detected in the T73 strain. Under these circumstances we can assume that, as in other S. cerevisiae strains, yeast DNA transfer can only be produced after cell breakage. Autolysis in *S. cerevisiae* begins after cells die, and during this process DNA is degraded before the cell wall is destroyed. As a result, release to the environment of intact free yeast DNA is unlikely.

Consumer safety

Following Roller and co-workers, in general the pathogenicity and potential toxicity of a genetically modified organism is governed by the pathogenicity or toxicity of the host organism, unless genes coding for virulence or toxin production have been used in the process of modifying the organism.[11] In the case of the recombinant T73 wine yeast strain, the foreign gene encodes an enzyme that cuts the internal bonds of cellulose molecules or its derivatives. It is difficult to conceive of any way this new phenotypic characteristic could transform the T73 strain to pathogenicity.

As additional comment, and in view of the review of the Gist-Brocades modified MAL-baker yeast, the UK Advisory Committee on Novel Foods and Processes has declared that there are no consumer safety reasons why the use of genetically modified yeast should not be permitted in foods.

Regulatory position of the recombinant wine yeast strain

To date, all fermentation with the recombinant T73 strains have been carried out as microvinification processes in sterile microbiological conditions. The wines produced have only been used for aroma testing and chromatographic analysis. Now it is necessary to carry out pilot plant experiments at the industrial level in order to confirm the results of the microvinifications and commercialize the "recombinant" wines.

The Spanish Biotechnology Law appeared a few weeks ago, on 3 June 1994.[12] The basic principle of this law is the protection of both human health and the natural environment. Following this legislation, we need to do the following:

1) We should petition the appropriate regional governmental body for permission to carry out the pilot plant experiments and present a complete scientific dossier detailing the procedure and assessment of the risks.

2) After one month, the regional government is required to present a report on the risks to the central government. At this time the central government sends this information to the EU, which then transmits the information to the other EU Member States. Objection by Member States must be notified to the regional government within three months.

3) If permission is obtained, the pilot plant fermentation will be carried out. It will be necessary to inform the regional government of the risks associated with the project.

4) The authorization for the commercialization of the "recombinant" wine will be obtained in a similar way, but in this case the appropriate administration is the central government.

Since this is a recent law, no clear responsibilities have been defined at the level of the regional governments. In fact, the Spanish government needs to create all the administrative instruments relating to this law before the end of the year.

Acknowledgements

The work at the IATA laboratory has been supported by a grant from the Commission Interministerial de Ciencia y Tecnología of the Spanish Government (ALI93-0809).

References

1. Querol, A., Huerta, T., Barrio, E. and Ramón, D. (1992) Dry yeast strain for use in fermentation of Alicante wines: selection and DNA patterns. *J. Food Sci.* 57:183-185, 216.

2. Querol, A., Barrio, E. and Ramón, D. (1992) A comparative study of different methods of yeast strain characterization. *System. Appl. Microbiol.* 15:439-446.

3. Querol, A., Barrio, E. and Ramón, D. (1994) Population dynamics of natural *Saccharomyces* strains during wine fermentation. *Int. J. Food Microbiol.* 21:315-323.

4. Querol, A., Barrio, E., Huerta, T. and Ramón, D. (1992) Molecular monitoring of wine fermentations conducted by active dry yeast strains. *Appl. Environ. Microbiol.* 58:2948-2953.

5. Ramón, D., Pérez-González, J.A., Barrio, E., González, R., Huerta, T., Sendra, J. and Querol, A. (1993) Molecular monitoring of wine fermentation. In: *Progress in Food Fermentation* Vol. 1 (Benedito de Barber et al., eds.). IATA, Valencia, pp. 324-329.

6. Pérez-González, J.A., González, R., Querol, A., Sendra, J. and Ramón, D. (1993) Construction of a recombinant wine yeast strain expressing β-(1,4)-endoglucanase and its use in microvinification processes. *Appl. Environ. Microbiol.* 59:2801-2806.

7. Günata, Y.Z., Bayonove, C.L., Baumes, R.L. and Cordonnier, R.E. (1985) The aroma of grapes. I. Extraction and determination of free and glycosidically bound fractions of some grape aroma components. *J. Chromatogr.* 331:83-90.

8. Günata, Y.Z., Dugelay, I., Sapis, J.C., Baumes, R.L. and Bayonove, C.L. (1990) Action des glycosidases exogènes au cours de la vinification : liberation de l'arôme à partir des précurseurs glycosidiques. *J. Int. Sci. Vignes Vin.* 24:133-144.

9. Vallés, S., Piñaga, F., Gallego, M.V. and Ramón, D. Manuscript in preparation.

10. González, R., Ramón, D. and Pérez González, J.A. (1992) Cloning, sequence analysis and yeast expression of the *egl1* gene from *Trichoderma longibrachiatum*. *Appl. Microbiol. Biotechnol.* 38:370-375.

11. Roller, S., Praaning-van Dalen, D. and Andreoli, P. (1994) The environmental implications of genetic engineering in the food industry. In: *Food Industry and the Environment* (J.M. Dalzell, ed). Blackie Academic and Professional, London, pp. 48-75.

12. Ley 15/1994 (1994) BOE 133, pp. 17781-17788.

Safety Approaches to Pure Culture Fermentation of Vegetables

Antonio de Castro

Instituto de la Grasa CSIC
Seville, Spain

Introduction

Fermented plant products are considered by many food scientists as "food of the future" (Buckenhüskes, 1993). Historically, fermentation has played an important role in providing safe, nutritious, and preserved vegetables. With the introduction of new techniques, such as freezing and canning, fermentation as a preservation method has become less important in developed countries. However, fermentation remains an important technology because it provides unique organoleptic qualities in the products, and allows the processing season of fruits and vegetables to be extended over a longer period of time. On the other hand, fermentation is still a primary method of vegetable preservation in developing countries, where it is a cheap, safe, and easy way to keep raw materials (Fleming and McFeeters, 1981).

There are many different fermented vegetables throughout the world. In fact, almost every plant product can be fermented in one way or another. The importance of each product is, in some instances, very limited to local markets, although with a high socioeconomic incidence. However, in Western Europe three products are of real economic importance: olives, sauerkraut and cucumbers. As an example, the production of table olives in 1992/93 was 1,017,000 tonnes, of which 200,000 tonnes was traded internationally (Anonymous, 1994).

Although not all table olives and cucumbers are fermented, those which are lactic acid-fermented constitute the most important products. The processes for manufacturing lactic acid-fermented vegetables vary, depending on the characteristics desired in the final product. Nevertheless, a generalized summary of the fermentation step can be made. Fresh vegetables, like most plant material, contain a numerous and varied epiphytic microflora including many potential spoilage microorganisms, and a small population of lactic acid bacteria. When vegetables are brined, fermentation occurs through a sequence of various types of microorganism. This sequence may be categorized into four stages: initiation, primary fermentation, secondary fermentation, and post-fermentation (**Table 1**) (Fleming and McFeeters, 1981).

It can be seen that an extraordinary complexity arises. Furthermore, lactic acid bacteria responsible for the natural fermentation of vegetables include the genera *Enterococcus*, *Leuconostoc*, *Pediococcus* and *Lactobacillus*, with *Lactobacillus plantarum* the most important species.

Table 1
Sequence of Microorganisms During Natural Fermentation of Brined Vegetables

Stage	Prevalent microorganisms
Initiation	Various Gram-negative and Gram-positive bacteria including *Enterobacteriaceae* and clostridia
Primary fermentation	Lactic acid bacteria and yeasts
Secondary fermentation	Yeasts
Post-fermentation	Spoilage might occur through surface-growing yeast and moulds or anaerobic growth of propionibacteria and clostridia if allowed

In addition, numerous chemical and physical factors influence rate and extent of growth of each microorganism and its sequence of appearance. These factors include, for example, acidity, pH and buffer capacity, salt concentration, temperature, natural inhibitory compounds, chemical additives, amount of fermentable carbohydrates and other nutrients in vegetable, etc.

It is also important to note that for some products without any heat treatment, various lactic acid bacteria and yeasts are still present at the moment of consumption.

Taking this complexity into account, it is not surprising that pure culture fermentation of vegetables is considered by most researchers in the area as the main goal to be achieved, in order to:

1) homogenize the final product;

2) prevent spoilage;

3) increase nutritive value and general quality; and

4) reduce salt content in wastewater.

To date, pure lactic starter cultures have not been very common in vegetable fermentations, although there are preparations on the market. Besides technological and economic factors, the lack of widespread commercial use of cultures is due to the fact that no strains are currently available which fulfill the desired requirements. In other words, although the development of improved controlled fermentation methods for vegetables is possible, commercial acceptance will depend on the development of better cultures and suitable tanking and handling procedures to make such methods economically attractive.

The ideal vegetable inoculant

Every product has its own peculiarities. However, a general description of the ideal traits is possible (**Table 2**) (Daeschel and Fleming, 1984; Buckenhüskes, 1993).

To find a single strain of lactic acid bacteria which meets all these attributes may seem impossible at present, but it is not impossible to acquire the necessary knowledge with that aim.

The genetics of lactobacilli are in their infancy. However, in the last few years rapid progress has been made, increasing our understanding to the point where manipulation is now possible. At the same time, improvements are being made in the understanding of the fermentation processes, as well as in the isolation of naturally occurring lactic acid bacteria with advantageous traits.

Current situation

The development of a suitable starter culture system is the first step in further investigation of fermentation with improved strains. For sauerkraut and cucumber, filter-sterilized juices have been used as model systems (Harris et al., 1992; Daeschel et al., 1988). A method for controlled fermentation of Spanish-type green olives has also been developed (Montaño et al., 1993). Furthermore, a dialysis pure-culture process for lactic acid fermentation of vegetables is available (Costilow and Gerhardt, 1983). However, enormous work remains to be done with regard to the metabolic capacities of the lactic acid bacteria strains involved in vegetable fermentations. A survey of some of the above mentioned traits can be made.

First of all, we look for a rapid and predominant growth. This will depend, of course, on the combined effect of all the intrinsic and extrinsic factors of each particular environment, with salt and acid contents as key variables. In fact, the final lactic acid concentration reached by *Lactobacillus plantarum* in cucumber juice will depend, among other factors, on the initial salt content (Passos et al., 1994).

Nowadays, greater salt tolerance is required for bacteria used in cucumber and olive fermentation (5-10 per cent salt) than in sauerkraut fermentation (0.6-2 per cent). However, bearing in mind a future development of pure culture fermentations, the salt content could be reduced if the texture retention is guaranteed.

By so doing, we will get two very important consequences: firstly, a reduction in the sodium intake of consumers; and secondly, a reduction in the salt content of the wastewater generated by the industry.

With regard to acid production and tolerance, rapid acid production is essential for lowering pH and inhibiting the growth of undesirable bacteria during fermentation. Furthermore, acid tolerance is necessary in order to remove all fermentable sugars and complete fermentation, preventing secondary fermentation by yeasts. Although the acid tolerance of *Leuconostoc mesenteroides* and *Lactobacillus plantarum* (the main species in vegetable fermentation) has been studied (McDonald et al., 1990), further research into the mechanism maintaining pH gradient between, inside and outside the cells is necessary.

Table 2
Desirable Traits in the Ideal Starter Culture for Vegetable Fermentations

Present	Lacking
Rapid and predominant growth	
Acid production and tolerance	Ability to metabolize
Salt tolerance	Formation of dextrans
Growth at low temperatures	Pectinolytic activity
Tolerance to natural inhibitory compounds	Cellulolytic activity
Formation of bacteriocins	Antibiotic resistance
Antimicrobial activity against yeasts, clostridia and others	Formation of biogenic amines
Bacteriophage resistance	Pathogenesis
Favourable nutritional effects	
Favourable sensorial effects	
Probiotic effects	

Besides antimicrobial activity, the acids produced during fermentation have an outstanding role in the sensorial and nutritional properties of the product. Heterofermentative lactic acid bacteria impart the characteristics desired in sauerkraut and olives (Montaño et al., 1993). In all cases, L-lactic acid isomer producer strains are preferred. On the other hand, the ability to metabolize organic acids is detrimental. Decarboxylation of malic acid is undesirable in cucumber fermentation because the CO_2 produced can contribute to bloater damage. A mutant strain of *Lactobacillus plantarum* without the ability to produce CO_2 from malate has been isolated (Daeschel et al., 1984).

This is probably the first instance in which a lactic acid bacterium has been genetically altered to obtain a specific metabolic trait desired in startercultures for fermented vegetables. *Lactobacillus plantarum* can even metabolize lactic acid anaerobically after prolonged incubation (Lindgren et al., 1990). If citrate is present together with glucose in the medium during the initial fermentation, the lactic and citric acid are degraded, resulting in the formation of formic, acetic and succinic acid.

It is clear that a considerable variation in end-products formation by *Lactobacillus plantarum* can be achieved, depending on substrate, cultivation conditions, and metabolic properties of the strains. By manipulating these factors, the desired compounds in the final product could be obtained.

The formation of bacteriocins and other antimicrobial compounds by lactic acid bacteria is today a subject of general interest. These substances are important not only as a desirable trait for starter cultures, but also as a possibility for the development of safe food preservatives. Many strains of lactic acid bacteria have been found to produce bacteriocins (De Vuyst and Vandamme, 1994; Hoover and Steenson, 1994) and some of them have been tested in various types of food fermentation. In the case of vegetables, a paired starter culture system for sauerkraut, consisting of a nisin-resistant *Leuconostoc mesenteroides* strain and a nisin-producing *Lactococcus lactis* strain, has been developed as a model although this system has not yet been studied in natural fermentations (Harris et al., 1992). More recently, a *Lactobacillus plantarum* strain, which produces two different bacteriocins, has been used successfully in natural fermentation of green olive (Ruiz-Barba et al., 1994). It has been demonstrated that the ability to produce bacteriocins confers a decisive advantage over the naturally occurring microflora.

Acid production and tolerance, and the formation of bacteriocins, are probably the main traits for the ideal vegetable inoculant. It is not possible in this presentation to make an extensive survey of all the above mentioned desirable traits – just to emphasize that although much research needs to be done on many subjects (for instance, nutritional, sensorial and probiotic effects), the development of strains of lactic acid bacteria capable of improving the properties of fermented vegetables seems to be a reasonable goal. At the same time, this improvement will require a better knowledge of the genetics of lactic acid bacteria useful for fermenting vegetables, which are far less well known than those of dairy lactic acid bacteria.

Genetic engineering for introducing new attributes into a given host will require the following (Goodman and Warner, 1992):

1) suitable substrate DNA encoding the characteristic to be introduced;

2) cloning vectors, plasmid or bacteriophage DNA molecules into which foreign DNA can be introduced, and which can be stably maintained by the host bacterium or facilitate introduction of the foreign genes into its chromosome;

3) methods of introducing these molecules into the host and selecting for their presence; and

4) a method of expressing the foreign gene product.

Provided sufficient research is carried out, genetically manipulated lactic acid bacteria have real potential. The idea that they could be designed for a particular product, problem or necessity is an attractive one. A bank of inoculants could be prepared and marketed to meet industrial requirements.

Safety of pure culture-fermented vegetables

Natural lactic acid fermentation of vegetables has proven its safety since prehistoric times. It is the use of genetically manipulated strains that needs to be proven safe, or rather not unsafe.

The theoretical risks associated with genetically manipulated microorganisms (WHO, 1991) could be grouped as:

1) dissemination of the microorganism in the environment, with a risk of upsetting environmentally balanced situations;

2) transmission of the recombinant genes to other microorganisms;

3) unintentional modification of the host genome, with alteration of any pathogen or toxic activity.

Governments, consumer groups and industry look for absolute results. They would like a scientific consensus on zero risk. Obviously, there is no absolute guarantee of safety. However, it is possible to develop different systems to make the risk as low as possible.

Dissemination of the microorganisms in an open system – and, at present, vegetable fermentations are open systems – may occur, but it must be remembered that pathogenic bacteria are continually being released in sewage effluent and are therefore handled and managed efficiently most of the time. Nevertheless, the survival rates of the manipulated organisms in a range of conditions likely to occur in the release area must be studied, as must the reproduction rate in the environment.

The risk of transmission of the recombinant genes to other microorganisms can be reduced. Ideally, the recombinant genes should be chromosomally integrated to reduce the likelihood of transfer, but safe plasmid systems could also be developed. It might be possible to engineer a plasmid so that it survives in its intended host but not in any other to which it may be transferred – a so-called suicide function.

With regard to unintentional modifications of the host genome, the best safety status could be reached if all the DNA were well-characterized.

In summary, both the possibility and need of research for improving strains of lactic acid bacteria to be used in vegetable fermentation are clear.

The real problem arises, as always, from the standpoint of economy. Considering all the kinds of risk (not only safety) and benefits associated with the subject we are dealing with, in one pan of the scales are the bulk of investments necessary for research on the following topics:

1) the physiology, metabolism and genetics of lactic acid bacteria;

2) the role of microorganisms in the nutritional, sensorial and probiotic properties of fermented vegetables; and

3) last but not least, research on how to assess the risk associated with the use of genetically manipulated microorganisms in food fermentation.

In the other pan of the scales, and in the most optimistic way possible, might be the presentation of these new products. They are called Bio-Veg, a lactic acid bacteria fermented vegetable blend. Their ingredients are cabbages, cauliflowers, carrots, cucumbers, olives (whatever vegetables you want), fermenting brine, and genetically modified starter cultures. They are nutritious, safe, wholesome, and delicious – rich in L-lactic acid, fibre, vitamins and amino acids, and lacking nitrates, nitrites and biogenic amines. And their periodic intake reduces the serum level of cholesterol, reduces the incidence of colon cancer, stimulates the immune response, promotes resistance to colonization by pathogens, and alleviates both diarrhoea and constipation.

They would be nice products but it is obvious that the research necessary for that hypothetical goal will never come from the modest margins of vegetable manufacturing companies. Public funds are absolutely necessary to carry out the studies mentioned above, particularly safety assessment studies.

Whether we will be able to achieve safe use of genetically manipulated microorganisms in food production or not, only the future can say. In our opinion, their acceptance by the consumer will be possible only if the compensation is truly outstanding.

References

Anonymous (1994) *Olivae* 50:12-15.

Buckenhüskes, H.J. (1993) Selection criteria for lactic acid bacteria to be used as starter cultures for various food commodities. *FEMS Microbiol. Rev.* 12:253-272.

Costillow, R.N. and Gerhardt, P. (1983) Dialysis pure-culture process for lactic-acid fermentation of vegetables. *J. Food Sci.* 48:1632-1636.

Daeschel, M.A. and Fleming, H.P. (1984) Selection of lactic acid bacteria for use in vegetable fermentations. *Food Microbiol.* 1:303-313.

Daeschel, M.A., McFeeters, R.F., Fleming, H.P., Klaenhammer, T.R. and Sanozky, R.B. (1984) Mutation and selection of *Lactobacillus plantarum* strains that do not produce carbon dioxide from malate. *Appl. Environ. Microbiol.* 47:419-420.

Daeschel, M.A., Fleming, H.P. and McFeeters, R.F. (1988) Mixed culture fermentation of cucumber juice with *Lactobacillus plantarum*m and yeasts. *J. Food Sci.* 53:862-864.

De Vuyst, L. and Vandamme, E.J. (eds.) (1994) *Bacteriocins of Lactic Acid Bacteria. Microbiology, Genetics and Applications.* Blackie Academic and Professional, London.

Fleming, H.P. and McFeeters, R.F. (1981) Use of microbial cultures: Vegetable products. *Food Technol.* 35:84-88.

Fleming, H.P., McFeeters, R.F. and Daeschel, M.A. (1985) The lactobacilli, pediococci, and leuconostoc: vegetable products. In: *Bacterial starter cultures for foods* (S.E. Gilliland, ed.). CRC Press, Boca Raton, Florida.

Goodman, S.A. and Warner, P.J. (1992) Prospects for the genetic manipulation of silage inoculants. Proceedings of the International Roundtable on Animal Feed Biotechnology. *Research and Scientific Regulation*, Agriculture Canada, Ottawa, pp. 121-132.

Harris, L.J., Fleming, H.P. and Klaenhammer, T.R. (1992) Novel paired starter culture system for sauerkraut, consisting of a nisin-resistant *Leuconostoc mesenteroides* strain and a nisin-producing *Lactococcus lactis*. *Appl. Environ. Microbiol.* 58:1484-1489.

Hoover, D.G. and Steenson, L.R. (eds.) (1994) *Bacteriocins of Lactic Acid Bacteria*. Academic Press, Inc., San Diego.

Lindgren, S.E., Axelsson, L.T. and McFeeters, R.F. (1990) Anaerobic L-lactate degradation by *Lactobacillus plantarum*. *FEMS Microbiol. Letters* 66:209-214.

McDonald, L.C., Fleming, H.P. and Hassan, H.M. (1990). Acid tolerance of *Leuconostoc mesenteroides* and *Lactobacillus plantarum*. *Appl. Environ. Microbiol.* 56: 2120-2124.

Montaño, A., Sanchez, A.H. and De Castro, A. (1993) Controlled fermentation of Spanish-type green olives. *J. Food Sci.* 58:842-844.

Passos, F.V., Fleming, H.P., Ollis, D.F., Felder, R.M. and McFeeters, R.F. (1994) Kinetics and modeling of lactic acid production by *Lactobacillus plantarum*. *Appl. Environ. Microbiol.* 60: 2627-2636.

Ruiz-Barba, J.L., Cathcart, D.P., Warner, P.J. and Jimenez-Diaz, R. (1994) Use of *Lactobacillus plantarum* LPCO 10, a bacteriocin producer, as a starter culture in Spanish-style green olive fermentations. *Appl. Environ. Microbiol.* 60:2059-2064.

WHO (1991) *Strategies for assessing the safety of foods produced by biotechnology*. World Health Organization, Geneva.

Demonstration of Safety: Myco-protein

P.J. Rodgers

Zeneca Bio Products
United Kingdom

In 1964, RHM Research Limited started a research programme aimed at the development of a novel human food based on the production of a filamentous fungus grown in continuous culture on a carbohydrate medium. In 1983, clearance for sale of the product, myco-protein, was given by the Ministry of Agriculture, Fisheries and Food (MAFF); in January 1985, products were launched in a supermarket in the UK. Sales in Western European countries have increased since that time. A detailed history of the development of the product and business is given in **Table 1**.

However, before any novel source of food could be introduced into the diet, it had to satisfy three basic requirements, namely it would:

1) be attractive to eat and be available at an acceptable price;

2) possess good nutritional properties;

3) be demonstrably safe to eat.

This paper describes the testing philosophy and the testing undertaken to demonstrate the safety of the product.

Definition, production and properties

The product developed was ultimately called "myco-protein" on the advice of the Food Advisory Committee in the UK. It is "a food derived from a filamentous fungus *Fusarium graminearum* (Schwabe), ATC 20334, and whose RNA content has been reduced."

The base myco-protein material is produced by a continuous fermentation process, shown diagrammatically in **Table 2**. Myco-protein at this stage is a "dough" containing around 25 per cent solids. The characterists and composition of myco-protein are shown in **Tables 3 and 4**.

Testing philosophy

When research started, the concept of testing the safety of a major food ingredient had not been developed to any great extent. Conventional toxicological testing based upon the principle of measuring the response in animals of feeding the test substance to determine a "no effect level" of 100 times the level of expected exposure or greater was obviously impossible. For interest, a comparison of philosophies of evaluation of food with discrete chemical entities is shown in **Tables 5 and 6**. However, it was necessary to demonstrate nutritional adequacy, absence of harm in a safety evaluation, and immunological adequacy, particularly the absence of allergenicity. A testing programme was therefore developed in which myco-protein was a major part of a test diet in an animal model.

Testing programme and findings

The prospect of testing a complex food material in high concentration without affecting the nutritional balance of a convenient laboratory diet was daunting and no doubt impossible. Therefore, semi-synthetic diets were constructed in which myco-protein supplied either all of the animals' protein requirement or half of the protein requirement, the other half supplied by casein. These diets were then compared to a diet in which all protein was supplied by casein, and to a conventional animal diet. The safety assessment was based upon the major responses (**Table 7**). The conclusions are shown in **Table 8**. Most of the animal studies were carried out using the rat as the test animal, although studies in baboons, rabbits and calves were also performed. Particular studies included one, three and six-month subchronic rat studies, a lifespan (with *in utero* phase) study in rats, a four-generation reproduction study in rats, and a teratology study in rats.

In summary, the results from these studies demonstrate the safety of the myco-protein when tested using an animal model. Such a testing programme, lasting about a decade, was not, however, without difficulty, mainly due to lack of knowledge and logistical problems; these are summarized in **Table 9**.

Toxicology and nutrition

As already stated, over-dosing with a major food component is impossible (although many of us try to do so from time to time) and hence semi-synthetic diets were chosen for safety assessment of myco-protein. It states the obvious to say that a high level of inclusion of a test material displaces something else from the conventional diet mix, and hence balancing of diet is critical. Failure to do so can lead to a multitude of problems which may be concluded to be toxicological in origin, whereas they are in reality caused by nutritional imbalance. The most commonly described is probably nephrocalcinosis.

Nutrition of the rat

This is not a well researched area, most animal nutrition information being available for "farm animals". Therefore, there has been a lack of available data for the composition of successful diets for lifespan and reproduction studies, a situation which has been alleviated by a publication in 1993 by the American Institute of Nutrition (AIN).[1]

Table 1
Historical Development

1964	Ranks Hovis Mcdougall started research, vision of Lord Rank
1968	Discovery of *Fusarium graminearum* (Schwabe), code name A3/5
1970	Studies of fermentation and nutritional profile
1972	Safety evaluation commenced
1978	Application to MAFF and discussions with MAFF/DoH
1980	Provisional approval to test-market
1983	Letter of approval to sell product
1985	Certificate of free sale issued by MAFF
	Partnership between RHM and ICI to develop business (Marlow Foods)
late 1980s/ early 1990s	Products also launched in Ireland, Holland, Belgium, Germany
1990	Marlow Foods becomes wholly-owned subsidiary of ICI (later subject to binary fission and owned by the ZENECA half)
to date	50 million packs sold; capacity for 14,000 tes pa

Table 2
Schematic Production Process

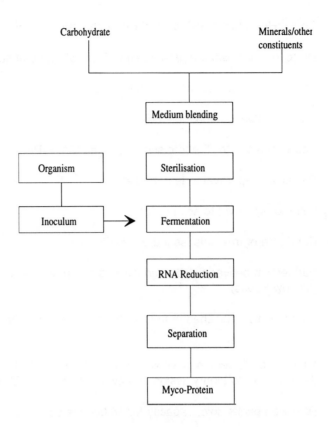

Table 3
Composition

	%
Crude protein TN x 6.25	55-60
True protein <u>a</u> aN X 6.22	45-50
RNA	< 2
Total lipid	12-13
Crude fibre	16-21
Dietary fibre	22-28
ASH	3-5

Table 4
Characteristics of Myco-protein

Good quality protein	:	45%+ protein on dry wt basis
	:	NPU greater than 85% of casein
High content of	:	25% on dry weight dietary fibre basis (mainly ß1,3,1,6-glucans, and chitin)
Low fat	:	13% on dry weight basis
Low sodium	:	200 mg/kg

No cholesterol

Can be textured due to filamentous structure

Buff-coloured, faint mushroom aroma

Table 5
Philosophy of Safety Evaluation

> For most drugs, agrochemicals and additives, evaluation is of chemicals of known composition, with clearly defined physical and chemical properties, usually at a low level of inclusion.
>
> Food, on the other hand, is a complex mixture which is consumed at a higher level of inclusion.
>
> The convention for evaluation to give a 100% margin of safety is impossible.

Table 6
Differences Between Chemical and Food Toxicity Evaluation

Chemical	Food
Material usually simple, chemically precise substance	Complex mixture of many compounds
Highest dose level should (and is indeed necessary to) produce an effect	Nutrition effects improbable; if seen, don't have a product
Small dose (usually less than 1% of diet)	High intake (usually greater than 10%)
Easy to give excessive dose	Over-consumption difficult
Acute effects often obvious	Acute effects difficult to produce (usually absent)
Generally independent of nutrition	Nutrition dependent
Specific route of metabolism simple to follow	Complex metabolism
Cause/effect relatively clear	Cause/effect may be confused

Table 7
Safety Assessment

Acute toxicity

Chronic toxicity

Carcinogenic potential

Effect on reproduction

Teratogenicity

Immunological effects

Table 8
Conclusions of the Safety Evaluations

- No potential toxicological effects in laboratory studies

- No dose-related adverse effects

- No anti-nutritional effects seen

- Analysis showed no unusual nitrogenous compounds

- Human nutritional studies indicated source of good-quality protein

- No major toxic effects identified from ingestion of myco-protein by humans

- No evidence of allergic reaction in volunteers

**Table 9
Difficulties "en route"**

- Difficulties many and varied:

    · toxicology vs. nutrition

    · lack of knowledge of nutrition of the rat

    · public perception

    · palatability/acceptability

    · foods generally moist, difficult for long-term studies

    · amount of material and consistency

    · dust

    · maternal/littering behaviour

- Obtaining myco-toxin free components of the diet

Public perception

Animal testing is a sensitive issue, regarded with concern by a number of people who have firmly held views. For a product such as myco-protein, which is seen as a potential alternative to the consumption of animal flesh, the fact that animal testing has been performed to satisfy regulatory and moral requirements is regarded as a counterbalancing feature.

Palatability/acceptability

A lifespan study, as the name implies, is for the lifetime of an animal. Any diet must therefore be acceptable for consumption by the animal for its lifetime, and must not cause any problems in its own right. For example, a "hard" diet can cause teeth to wear out, a dusty diet causes blocked nasal passages, and for some animals the boredom of lack of variety causes loss of appetite. Diet therefore has to be formulated from ingredients and prepared and presented in a physical form, such that it is acceptable and palatable to animals in the long term and does not cause any effect due to its consumption.

Moisture content

Myco-protein is typical of many foods. It has a relatively high moisture content, ca 70-75 per cent. The feeding of a moist diet over a long period of time is a major logistical problem, which cannot be overcome without very significant expense. Therefore, a case has to be presented on the equivalence of feeding an essentially "dry" diet.

Quantities

A lifespan study typically requires ca 2 1/2 tes of diet per test group (i.e. 10 tes for study) and a reproduction study 1 tes per test group. These are required over a two-year period, and there is a requirement to demonstrate consistency over that period. This necessitates a high level of supervision and analytical data. The number of diet suppliers who can produce to the "quality standards" required is limited.

Dust/maternal/littering behaviour

Dustiness of semi-synthetic diet can be a major problem causing breathing difficulties, particularly in small animals. Maternal behaviour also varies. Use of the diet to build a nest is not uncommon, and this can then lead to dust on the skin of newborns, causing dehydration as well as breathing difficulties.

Myco-toxin free diet

There have been concerns expressed about the ability of *Fusarium* to produce myco-toxins and hence pose a hazard to human health. In reality, the component of diet which we have been able to demonstrate to be free of myco-toxin has been myco-protein. However, obtaining other components of diet to the same high standards has proved difficult.

Immunological effects

During the research and development phase of the project, production workers exposed to the material were monitored for any immunological response and trials were carried out on human volunteers who had consumed the product. During testing, some 4500 individuals consumed the material and only one positive response was observed. The person concerned exhibited nausea, sickness and stomach pains, but was normal in 24 hours. Further tests indicated a sensitive atopic who had a cross-reaction to other fungal species. Monitoring of the product post-launch has led to people who had made complaints of illness following consumption of product volunteering to attend hospital and be tested by a skin prick test and measurement of RAST. This study yielded largely negative results, and led to the conclusion that no significant immunological problem arises from consumption of myco-protein.

Nutritional quality

In addition to toxicological studies a number of studies were conducted, prior to product launch, to demonstrate the nutritional quality of the product. The studies conducted and the results are summarized in **Tables 10 and 11**.

Following launch of the product a number of studies on the influence of myco-protein consumption on blood cholesterol levels and on satiety have been made. These indicated that consumption of myco-protein can make a positive contribution to a "balanced diet" and what is regarded in the 1990s as a "healthy diet".

Consumer experience

Safety testing *does not* end with the animal testing programme, and a complaints and follow-up procedure is maintained by the business. This indicates that in nearly a decade of trading the number of complaints is to be 1-1.5 per million products sold. This compares favourably with existing products in the marketplace. Investigation into complaints of ill-health have established no positive relationship to the product, and are in fact less than the incidence of reported ill-health in the population.

Conclusions

After over a decade of detailed investigation, the results were submitted to and considered by the Ministry of Agriculture Fisheries and Food (MAFF). Clearance was given to market the product in 1983 and a Certificate of Free Sale issued in 1985. The product has been on sale in Western Europe since then, and data from the marketplace indicates acceptability and absence of safety problems.

Acknowledgement

The author wishes to thank G.L. Solomons, D.G. Edwards and G.H. Pigott for the major contributions made by them over many years, without which this paper could not have been prepared.

Table 10
Measurement of Nutrition Value

Study	Assay	Animal species
Protein quality	digestibility NPU PER slope ratio available amino acids, e.g. lysine, methionine	rats rats rats rats chicks, rats
Energy	digestible	chicks, rats
Availability	metabolizable	chicks, rats
Trace nutrients	vitamins and minerals	chicks, rats, etc.
Feeding trials	various	rats, chickens, pigs, calves, etc.

Table 11
Nutrition Values for MCP

A.	Animal trials		
a)	Rat assays	NPU	PER
	MCP	61	2.4
	MCP and methionine	82	2.4
	Casein	70	2.5
b)	Chick assay Metabolizable energy	3.0 Kcal/g	
B.	Human studies		
b)	Human study	Biological value	
	MCP	84	
	Milk protein	85	

Food Safety Assessment of Transgenic Insect-resistant Bt tomatoes

H.A. Kuiper and H.P.J.M. Noteborn

State Institute for Quality Control of Agricultural Products
Department of Risk Assessment and Toxicology
The Netherlands

Introduction

Application of genetic engineering techniques in agriculture has resulted in the introduction of specific traits in a crop plant like for instance insect and virus resistance, cold/drought resistance, herbicide tolerance and delayed ripening of fruits. Characterization of the safety of genetically modified foods for the consumer is a topic of concern, and during the last few years various test strategies have been proposed by national governments and international organisations.[1] Although differences may be noted between proposed test strategies, a general agreement is noticed concerning the need for research of the introduced gene/products and the possibilities of secondary changes in the host organism as a result of gene modification.

In 1991, an EU co-sponsored research project was initiated in the framework of FLAIR (Food-linked Agro-Industrial Research) entitled *Opportunities of transgenic food crops for the consumer and the food industry in the Community*, with the objective to design a test strategy for the food safety evaluation of genetically modified foods. The project concerns the molecular/biochemical and toxicological characterization of tomato transformants genetically modified by the introduction of a gene encoding an insecticidal crystal protein, CRYIA(b), from *Bacillus thuringiensis*. Furthermore, an easily detectable marker gene, encoding for neomycin phosphotransferase (NPTII) is co-introduced into the plant genome for selection purposes.

Partners in the project are Plant Genetic Systems N.V., Ghent, Belgium (co-ordinator); the State Institute for Quality Control of Agricultural Products (RIKILT-DLO), Wageningen, the Netherlands, in co-operation with the Department of Toxicology of the Agricultural University of Wageningen, and with the Department of Environmental Sciences of the University La Tuscia, Viterbo, Italy; SME Ricerche SCPA, La Fagianeria, Piana di Monte Verna, Italy, and the University of Genova, DIBE, Genova, Italy. Results of the food safety studies of Bt tomatoes have been reported at various international meetings.[2-5]

Experimental strategy

The strategy for the evaluation of the food safety of the transgenic Bt tomato has been designed on the basis of the following considerations:

1) Does the introduced Bt protein exert toxic effects in mammals similar to the ones observed in target insect species? It is known that the insecticidal activity of CRYIA protein on larvae of *Lepidoptera* insects occurs through binding to specific membrane receptors present in epithelial midgut cells, leading to a disruption of potassium and sodium gradients and cell lysis.[6-9] Specific *in vivo* and *in vitro* studies have therefore been carried with recDNA CRYIA(b) produced in *E. coli*, in order to search for the presence of Bt receptors in mammalian tissues (including human) and possible histopathological damage.

2) Do the newly introduced proteins cause general systemic toxic effects in mammals, in particular immunotoxic (allergenic) effects? *In vitro* and *in vivo* studies have been carried out to investigate the digestibility of the newly introduced proteins and the systemic toxic potency upon oral administration to rodents.

3) Does genetic modification to tomato lines lead to significant changes in the nutritional composition of the modified tomato, or in the content of naturally occurring toxicants, which could negatively influence the safety of the product for the consumer? To this end comparative analytical studies have been carried out on the composition of macro and micro nutrients of modified tomatoes and the classical counterpart. Furthermore, a 90-day feeding trial has been performed with transgenic tomatoes as part of a rat diet, in order to test for unintended adverse effects of the genetically modified food.

Test materials

Transgenic tomato plants were obtained from different parental lines (TL001 a round type tomato, and SM002 a cylindrical elongated type) by *Agrobacterium tumefaciens* mediated transformation. These experiments have been carried out at Plant Genetic Systems. Details of the methodology are described in references 10-13. The transformation vector contained two chimeric genes coding for neomycin phosphotransferase II (NPTII), a marker gene, and the truncated Bt2 gene cloned from *B. thuringiensis* var. *berliner* 1715 coding for the protein CRYIA(b). Expression levels of CRYIA(b) protein in transgenic tomatoes varied between 7.5 ng/mg and 25.4 ng/mg of protein, while the levels of NPTII protein in ripe tomatoes were five to ten times higher.

In order to produce sufficient quantities for the toxicity and binding studies, recBt2 and recNPTII protein have been isolated and purified from *Escherichia coli* (K514) (11,14). Bt protein was subsequently digested with trypsin and chymotrypsin to yield the active toxic fragment CRYIA(b) (Mr 66-68 kDa).

Insecticidal activity of CryIA(b) in mammals

In male Brown Norway rats fed recCRYIA(b) protein in a quantity corresponding to a human daily consumption of approximately 2000 kg of transgenic Bt tomatoes, no binding of the CRYIA(b) protein could be observed in tissue segments of the g.i. tract. Immunocytochemical analysis of these tissues was performed using a polyclonal antiserum from rabbits. Furthermore, no histopathological damage has been detected, in contrast to what was observed in the brush border epithelium of the midgut of larvae of *Manduca sexta*.[14-16]

In vitro binding studies of recBt2 protein performed in intestinal tissue sections of rats, mice, Rhesus monkeys and humans, using monoclonal or polyclonal antisera from mouse or rabbits, also did not indicate specific binding of CRYIA(b) protein in contrast to binding in *Manduca sexta* larvae.

Digestibility of CRYIA(b) and of NPTII proteins

The digestibility of CRYIA(b) protein has been studied in male Brown Norway rats, fistulated in the ileum before the caecum. Animals were fed CRYIA(b) protein mixed with standard feed, in a quantity corresponding to a human daily consumption of 2000 kg transgenic Bt tomatoes. Chymus was collected after five to seven hours, and immunoblotting analysis revealed no intact protein, but fragments of 20-30 kDa and smaller. In samples taken after seven hours no larvae fragments of CRYIA(b) were visible, indicating a further extensive degradation of the protein during gastro-intestinal tract passage into smaller peptides with molecular weights << 9 kDa.

The degradation of CRYIA(b) protein and of NPTII has also been studied under simulating human gastro-intestinal conditions. Incubation of the proteins at pH 2 in the presence of pepsin, and subsequently at pH 8, in the presence of chymotrypsin and trypsin, revealed upon analysis by GPC and SDS-gel electrophoresis, followed by immunoblotting, an extensive fragmentation of the proteins to peptides with molecular weights below 10 kDa. The degradation of the CRYIA(b) protein is clearly a two-step process. After two hours at pH 2 in the presence of pepsin the protein was readily cleaved to yield a 15 kDa fragment, and successively to smaller fragments after continued treatment with chymotrypsin and trypsin at pH 8. The NPTII protein on the contrary appeared completely digested at pH 2 in the presence of pepsin.

Short-term Oral Toxicity Studies of CRYIA(b) in rodents

CRYIA(b) protein was orally dosed to female NMRI mice via drinking water *ad lib.* during 28 days. The highest dose level corresponded to a daily consumption of 500 kg of transgenic tomatoes. There were no differences observed in body weight gain, absolute and relative weights of liver and kidneys, and haematological parameters, including white blood cell differential counts, between treated and control animals. Furthermore, histopathological analysis of the gastro-intestinal tract of these animals did not reveal any adverse effects.

Studies have also been performed with CRYIA(b) protein administered to New Zealand White male rabbits via drinking water *ad lib.* during 31 days. Data of average water consumption indicated a daily intake of CRYIA(b) protein corresponding to a human daily consumption of 60 kg transgenic Bt tomatoes. There were no changes observed in food consumption and water intake nor in body weight gain and absolute and relative liver and kidney weights between treated and non-treated animals. No differences were noted in haematological parameters, including white blood cell differential counts. Furthermore, histological analysis of various segments of the gastro-intestinal tract did not reveal any harmful effects in the treated animals. Analysis of serum samples taken two and four weeks after initiation of the experiment, did not indicate that antibodies against CRYIA(b) were induced in treated animals. In immunoglobulin (IgG) content of the serum of treated animals compared to that of control animals.

Haemolytic potency of CRYIA(b) protein

Some varieties of Bt proteins may exert hemolytic effects, like Bt derived from *B. thuringiensis* SSP *israelensis*.[17] Therefore human red blood cells (RBC) were tested for the Haemolytic potential of CRYIA(b), by incubation of the RBCs with the protein, and monitoring the osmotic fragility by electron microscopy and spectroscopically. No haemolysis was observed. It has been postulated that the site of interaction of CRYIA(b) may be the ATPase, which is located on the cytoplasmatic side of the membrane of RBCs.[18] Therefore CRYIA(b) has been entrapped inside the RBC by the method of hypotonic dialysis,[19] and subsequently tested for its haemolytic potency. Erythrocytes containing CRYIA(b) showed negligible haemolysis comparable to that of control RBCs containing entrapped albumin.

Food Safety of transgenic Bt tomatoes

Chemical analysis of nutrients and glycoalkaloids

After field testing mature red tomatoes (the transgenic Bt tomato line RLE13-0009 and the non-transformed control line TL001) were harvested, and samples of freeze-dried material were analyzed for macro and micro nutrients. The contents of total protein, fat, carbohydrates, fiber, vitamin C, and minerals like calcium, phosphorus, chloride, sodium potassium, magnesium and iron were comparable between transformed Bt tomatoes and non-transformed ones, and were found to be within published ranges.[20]

No significant differences were observed in the concentrations of α-tomatine between mature tomatoes of modified plants and controls (range: 1.4-1.7 mg α-tomatine/kg fresh weight). Other known solanaceous alkaloids (i.e. solanine) were not detected.

91-day feeding trial with transgenic tomatoes

The field grown transgenic Bt tomato line RLE13-0009 and the control line TL001 have been tested in a 91-day feeding study in rats. The field trial manifested no significant differences in vegetative growth and harvest characteristics between transgenic Bt tomatoes and the controls. In the harvested transgenic tomato variety CRYIA(b) protein was typically expressed in fresh tomatoes (i.e. non-induced) at levels of 7.5 ng/mg protein.

Three groups of male and female weanling Wistar rats were fed during a period of 91 days respectively a control semi synthetic animal diet (Muracon SSP TOX), the same diet supplemented with 10 per cent (w/w) of lyophilized transgenic tomato material, containing 40.6 ng Bt protein/mg protein, or with 10 per cent (w/w) of lyophilized material from the control parent line. The macro- and micronutrient composition was equalized in all diets. The amounts of supplementary minerals and vitamins were deduced from the actual levels in freeze-dried tomatoes. The average daily intake of the diets over the 91 days period correspond to 200 g of tomatoes/kg body weight, equivalent to a daily human consumption of 13 kg tomatoes. There was no feed refusal or unusual behaviour observed in the animals. No significant differences have been noticed in survival, clinical signs, body weight, feed consumption, feed efficiency, absolute and relative organ weights, haematological values, and clinical chemistry parameters between the different diet groups, and no macroscopic abnormalities were found. Ig-antibody measurements in serum and microscopic histological analysis of organs and tissues is in progress.

Conclusions

Results obtained up till now indicate that:

1) No specific receptors for CRYIA(b) protein are present along the g.i. tract of mammals including man. Furthermore, no histopathological effects of the protein have been observed in the digestive mucosa cells lining the gastro-intestinal tract of mammals.

2) CRYIA(b) and NPTII degrade rapidly under simulating gastrointestinal conditions to smaller fragments with molecular weights below 10 kDa, and CRYIA(b) is upon high dosage oral feeding to rats digested extensively in the g.i. tract to smaller peptides.

3) CRYIA(b) orally administered to mice and rabbits, does not exert signs of systemic adverse effects. No indications were found for immunotoxic effects as judged from the histological examination of spleen, lymph nodes and the Peyer's patches of treated animals. Furthermore, in serum of treated rabbits no specific antibodies against CRYIA(b) protein could be detected, nor was the total IgG concentration elevated with respect to control animals. *In vitro* experiments to test for the haemolytic potency of the CRYIA(b) protein yielded negative results.

4) No major changes occur in the chemical composition of transgenic tomatoes as a result of the insertion of foreign genes. It should be noted that nutritional components of plants normally vary due to both cultivar-related and environmental influences. Moreover levels of the naturally occurring toxicant α-tomatine were similar in modified and control tomatoes.

5) Transgenic Bt tomatoes fed to rats during 91 days as lyophilized powder mixed through the diet, do not exert any signs of adverse effects. The estimated average intake of tomato powder during the test period corresponded to a daily human consumption of 13 kg of fresh tomatoes. Food intake, body and organ weights, and clinical parameters were normal and gross macroscopic examination of tissues did not indicate toxic effects. Histopathological analysis of organs and tissues is in progress. Although final conclusions cannot be drawn yet, the toxicological data obtained up till now are reassuring with respect to food safety of the modified Bt tomatoes.

Future work

A number of aspects concerning the food safety of transgenic Bt tomatoes has still to be studied:

1) Post-translational modifications: Studies performed up till now have been carried out with recDNA CRYIA(b) protein purified from *E. coli*. Differences in post-translation modifications in prokaryotic and eukaryotic systems (degree and kind of amidation, glycosylation, phosphorylation of proteins), may influence the toxic potential of introduced proteins.

2) Allergenic potency: The allergenic potency of the CRYIA(b) protein has not been tested. Although long term use of Bt crystal protein inclusions as a spray has not revealed evidence for allergenic reactions in workers, studies on the allergenic potency of the CRYIA(b) protein should be considered, in particular because of the potential general exposure of the population to CRY proteins via transgenic crop plants.

3) Secondary effects: Chemical analysis of naturally occurring toxicants in order to detect possible secondary metabolic changes in plants as a result of foreign gene insertion, has its limitations due to the lack of appropriate analytical methods. Therefore new ways of analysis should be explored, focusing at the characterization of plant extracts with respect to **"metabolite fingerprints"** rather than isolation and structural characterization of single compounds. This analytical approach may offer possibilities to limit animal feeding trials with whole foods.

Risk evaluation of transgenic food crops with respect to human consumption must be based on the specific genetic modifications involved, and the characteristics of introduced genes and expression products; furthermore attention should be paid to possible secondary metabolic changes occurring as a result of gene manipulation, and the level of potential exposure of the human population should be determined. Safety assessment of genetically modified foods should take place within a general framework with "case-by-case" variations, taking the often long history of safe use of traditional "counterpart" foods into account. Development of new analytical and *in vitro* toxicological methods offers interesting possibilities for the assessment of food safety aspects of transgenic crops.

Acknowledgements

We thank Dr B. Verachtert and Dr A. Reynaerts, Plant Genetic Systems, Ghent, Belgium, for provision and biochemical characterization of test materials and methods for their invaluable advice and stimulating collaboration. We thank Dr M. Pensa, SME Ricerche SCPA, Piana di Monte Verna, Italy, for providing transgenic and control tomatoes and for carrying out the compositional analysis of the tomatoes; Prof L. Zolla, University La Tuscia, Viterbo, Italy, for performing the hemolysis experiments; M. Peters and G. van Tintelen, Centre for Small Laboratory Animals of the Agricultural University, Wageningen, for their assistance with the animal experiments; Dr G.M. Alink and J.H.J. van den Berg, Department of Toxicology, Agricultural University, and Dr M.J. Groot and J.S. Ossekoppele, RIKILT-DLO, Wageningen, for their contribution to the gross and histological examination of test animals; M.E. Bienenmann-Ploum, J.F. Labrijn, G.J.M. Loeffen, G.D. van Bruchem, H.J. van Egmond, A. de Koning, A.R.M. Hamers, M.B.M. Huveneers-Oorsprong and H.M. van de Putte, RIKILT-DLO, for histological, clinical and chemical analysis. This work was carried out in the framework of the EU Food-Linked Agro-Industrial Research (FLAIR) program (Contract No. AGRF-CT90-0039).

References

1. Kok, E.J., Reynaerts, A. and Kuiper, H.A. (1993) *Trends in Food Science and Technology* 4:42-48.

2. Noteborn, H.P.J.M., Rienenmann-Ploum, M.E., van den Berg, J.H.J., Alink, G.M., Zolla, L. and Kuiper, H.A. (1993) Food safety of transgenic tomato expressing the insecticidal crystal protein CrylA(b) from *Bacillus thuringiensis* and the marker enzyme APH(3')II. *Med. Fac. Landbouww. Univ. Gent*, Vol. 58/4b, 1951-1858.

3. Noteborn, H.P.J.M., Rienenmann-Ploum, M.E., van den Berg, J.H.J., Alink, G.M., Zolla, L. and Kuiper, H.A. (1994) Consuming transgenic food crops: the toxicological and safety aspects of tomato expressing CrylA(b) and NPTII. In: *Proc. 6th European Congress on Biotechnology* (L. Alberghina, L. Frontali and P. Sensi, eds.). Elsevier Science B.V., 1045-1048.

4. Noteborn, H.P.J.M., Bienenmann-Ploum, M.E., Alink, G.M., Zolla, L. and Kuiper, H.A. (1994) Safety Assessment of Transgenic Tomato Fruit Expressing the Truncated Gene CrylA(b) from *Bacillus thuringiensis* subsp. *berliner 1715*. *Toxicology Letters* 74 (Suppl. 1), 58.

5. Noteborn, H.P.J.M., Bienenmann-Ploum, M.E., van den Berg, J.H.J., Alink, G.M., Zolla, L. and Kuiper, H.A., Safety assessment of the *Bacillus thuringiensis* insecticidal crystal protein CrylA (b) expressed in transgenic tomatoes. In: *Safety Aspects of Flavors and Foods Produced by Genetically Modified Plants and Organisms* (K.H. Engel, G. Takeoka and R. Teranshi, eds.). ACS Symposium Series (submitted).

6. Hendrickx, K., De Loof, A. and van Mellaert, H. (1990) *Comp. Biochem. Physiol.* 95C(2): 241-245.

7. Knowles, B.H. and Ellar, D.J. (1987) *Biochim. Biophys. Acta* 924:509-518.

8. Endo, Y. and Nishiitsutsuji-Umo, J. (1980) *Invertebr. Pathol.* 36:90-103.

9. Percy, J. and Fast, P.G. (1983) *J. Invertebr. Pathol.* 41:86-98.

10. Velten et al. (1984) *Embo J.* 3:2723-2730.

11. Beck, E., Ludwig, G., Auerswald, E., Reiss, B. and Schaller, H. (1982) *Gene* 327-336.

12. Gielen, J., Beuckeleer, M. de, Seurinck, J., Deboeck, F., Greve, H. de, Lemmers, M., Montagu, M. van and Schell, J. (1984) *Embo J.* 3:835-846.

13. Hain et al. (1985) *Mol. Gen. Genet.* 199:161-168.

14. Hoffmann, C., Vanderbruggen, H., Höfte, H., van Rie, J., Jansens, S. and van Mellaert, H. (1988) *Proc. Natl. Acad. Sci. USA* 85:7844-7848.

15. Van Rie, J., McGaughey, W.H., Johnson, D.E., Barnett, B.D. and van Mellaert, H. (1990) *Science* 2476:72-74.

16. Van Rie, J., Jansens, S., Höfte, H., Degheele, D. and van Mellaert, H. (1990) *Appl. Environ. Microbiol.* 56:1378-1385.

17. Gill, S.S., Singh, G.J.P. and Hornung, J.M. (1987) Cell membrane interaction of *Bacillus thuringiensis* Subsp. israelensis, cytolytic Toxins. *Infect. Immun.* 55:1300-1309.

18. English, L.H. and Cantley, L.C. (1986) *J. Biol. Chem.*, 261:1170-1173.

19. Zolla, L., Lupidi, G., Marcheggiani, M., Falcioni, G. and Brunori, M. (1990) *Biochim. Biophys. Acta* 1024:1-9.

20. *Food Composition and Nutrition Tables 1986/1987* (1986) (S.W. Souci, W. Fachmann and H. Kraut, eds.). Wissenschaftliche Verlagsgesellschaft mbH, Stuttgart, 694-695.

Evaluation of Toxicological Studies on Flavr Savr Tomato

David Hattan

United States Food and Drug Administration

Recently (1994), the FDA approved the marketing of a new variety of delayed ripening tomato, the Flavr Savr tomato. This new strain was developed using recombinant DNA technology to insert an antisense DNA that resulted in a very significant reduction in the expression of the polygalacturonase enzyme, responsible for the softening of the fruit. This reduced concentration of softening enzyme allows the fruit to remain longer on the vine before harvesting and also provides some extension of shelf life for the fruit once sent to market.

While engaged in the process of acquiring the necessary evidence to support the safety of the new Flavr Savr transgenic strain of tomatoes, Calgene appropriately characterized the nature and extent of the genetic materials transferred to the new tomato was: fa full length copy of the appropriate gene, the construct was well described and characterized, no contaminating proteins were encoded by extraneous, uncharacterized DNA, and there were no gene-sized DNA fragments or transformable DNA in the enzyme preparation.

In addition the company established that there was no decrement in the concentration of normal nutrients (vitamin A,C, Bs, magnesium, calcium or phosphorus) and there was no augmentation of the level of toxicants (tomatine) in this genetically modified strain of tomato.

As an added measure of assurance of the safety of this new variety of tomatoes, Calgene contracted with the International Research and Development Corporation (IRDC) for the conduct of three studies in experimental animals. The three studies were conducted by IRDC in six-week old male and female rats supplied by Charles River that were gavaged with either deionized water, control (non-transgenic) or transgenic (Flavr Savr) tomatoes for 28 days. The first two materials serving as vehicle and tomato controls, respectively, for the latter or test group.

This type of acute, multidose toxicological study is normally conducted to assess whether there are any major types of adverse effects manifested during administration of the test material. The major effects monitored or measured usually include food consumption, body weight gain, organ weights, hematology and clinical chemistry and not uncommonly there is also an assessment of potential direct organ system toxicity by histopathological analysis of tissues. In all three of these 28-day studies comparable results were obtained regarding major indicators of toxicity referred to in the preceding paragraph. Comparison of gross and microscopic histopathological results from this study revealed no difference in the occurrence of tissue abnormalities between the water control group, the non-transgenic tomato control group and the transgenic test group.

In the first study however, Calgene supplied to IRDC for test administration a strain of transgenic tomato that was not utilized for commercial purposes. Thus, IRDC subsequently completed a second 28-day gavage study in rats gavaged with a water control, separate groups gavaged with two different strains of transgenic tomato that Calgene intended to sell to consumers and a fourth treatment group that received tomatoes from a non-transgenic strain. During postmortem evaluation, grossly visible stomach lesions were found in 4 of 20 female rats given one of the transgenic tomatoes but not in the other three groups of treated rats. For each of the four treatment groups included in this study, all major parameters described above were within normal limits for this strain of rats.

Calgene then decided to conduct a third 28-day gavage study to try to clarify whether the effect observed in the one transgenic strain of tomatoes in the second study was replicable and uniquely attributable to this transgenic strain of tomatoes, This third study was performed with four treatment groups of rats; animals receiving water as a control, those receiving transgenic tomato (the strain in which the effect on the stomach had been observed), those given the same transgenic tomato but grown in another geographic location and a group of rats that received treatment with a non-transgenic tomato strain. In an effort to assess whether the stomach erosion effect was replicable and dose-responsive, the third study included additional treatment groups in the non-transgenic and transgenic tomato test groups that received even greater doses of tomato than in the previous two studies.

Again, as in the second study, the only evidence of adverse effect was found following gross and microscopic histopathological examination of the stomach. The same type of relatively minor erosions were found. However, in this particular study, the stomach effects were found to occur more widely, in eight of eleven treatment groups. While the actual numerical incidence of stomach erosions diagnosed from the microscopic histopathology slides by two different pathology groups were slightly different as reported by Calgene, the overall analysis was common to both pathology groups, i.e. that the stomach erosions observed in these studies were incidental and not correlated specifically and/or consistently with any treatment group, including the transgenic tomato-treated groups.

Assessment

In the process of evaluating the results from this type of acute study, it is important to remember the class of effects normally monitored. the 28-day study is typically used to determine whether any major adverse changes have been observed in the experiment. Parameters usually assessed are food consumption, body weight changes, comparative effects on organ weights, clinical chemistry and hematology and histopathology. With respect to these indicators of major adverse effect, there were no differences observed either between treatment groups within a given study or across the three studies. the one possible exception to this conclusion is a possible difference in comparative histopathological effects on the stomach. As reported by Calgene, there was no difference in the rate of occurrence of stomach erosions in rats assigned to a given type of treatment even when the dose of tomato was doubled as in the third gavage study. Moreover, Calgene's report of the histopathology of the stomach indicated that when one compared histopathology results across studies, there was no overall change in the morphology or increased severity of the stomach erosions. Additionally, due to the variable and inconsistent observation of the stomach erosions across studies, it is not clear that there was any true treatment-related effect.

Historically, any studies that have been conducted to assess the toxicity of a whole food have been fraught with inherent limitations in the study protocols (Hattan, 1994; Hammond, 1994). Unlike more potent and typical food additives, it is not possible to effectively exaggerate the dose of test material administered when assessing the potential toxicity of a whole food without increasing the likelihood of introducing confounding effects in the study, e.g. nutritional incompatibilities. In the toxicological testing of irradiated foods, for example, it eventually became clear that using too high a concentration of whole food in the diet of experimental animals simply resulted in a high probability of adverse effects that were attributable to induced nutritional effects that were inadvertently manifested and not caused by a direct toxic effect of the test material (Hattan, 1994).

In the present instance of the transgenic tomato, the conclusion that seems best to account for the effects observed is that if there is a treatment-related effect, it is not unique to the transgenic strain of tomato and is more likely to be simply a physiological response to uncontrolled environmental stressors, such as protracted fasting, changes in room temperature, or handling of animals during gavage. Alternatively it is possible that the relatively minor changes observed in stomach lining morphology in these studies are the result of the ingestion by the rats of very large quantities of tomato and thus are not uniquely attributable to the transgenic strain of tomatoes. It is unusual for a gavage dose (15 ml twice daily) to be administered to an animal. The National Toxicology Program uses 5 ml per single gavage dose as the maximum in its testing program. In a recent study submitted to the FDA on another food additive material, the dose utilized was 10ml per single gavage dose and likely because of the large dose and possible other technical difficulties with dose administration, the study had to be cancelled due to mortality. When the study was restarted with smaller injection volumes, the study was completed successfully.

References

Hammond, B. "Limitations of Whole Food Feeding Studies in Food Safety Assessment" (this Workshop).

Hattan, D. G. "Lessons Learned from the Toxicological Testing of Irradiated Foods" (this Workshop).

Safety Evaluation of Glyphosate-tolerant Soybeans

**Roy L. Fuchs,[1] Diane B. Re, Steve G. Rogers,
Bruce G. Hammond and Stephen R. Padgette**

The Agricultural Group, Monsanto
United States

Introduction

Numerous genetically engineered plant products have been extensively field tested and are moving towards market introduction. The first of these products, the Flavr-Savr™ tomato, was recently introduced in the United States after lengthy consultations with the United States Food and Drug Administration. Confirming the safety and satisfying the appropriate regulatory agencies are key steps in the development of these products. A case study using soybeans that have been modified to be tolerant to glyphosate (glyphosate-tolerant soybeans, GTS) will be used to illustrate the detailed technical assessment employed to establish that these soybeans are substantially equivalent to the soybeans in commerce today.

We have carefully followed the guidance provided by both the Organization for Economic Cooperation and Development (OECD, 1993) and the Food and Drug Administration (US FDA, 1992) in assessing the safety of GTS. This assessment, which focused on the composition and nutrition of soybeans and the safety of the introduced protein that confers glyphosate tolerance, leads to the conclusion that GTS are substantially equivalent to the soybeans currently in commerce. Detailed compositional analysis of several other genetically engineered crops will be presented to verify that many of the genetically engineered crops being developed are substantially equivalent to the corresponding products currently marketed.

Background on glyphosate-tolerant soybeans

Weed control in agricultural crops is critical to maintain yield, harvest efficiency, seed quality and eliminate weeds that serve as a reservoir for crop pests. Today, nearly 100 per cent of the corn and soybeans grown in the United States are treated with herbicides (Gianessi et al., 1991). New weed control systems are needed to provide improved weed control and greater application flexibility, to provide alternative modes-of-action for more effective weed management systems and to provide herbicides with enhanced environmental characteristics. New herbicides have typically been discovered by extensive screening to evaluate not only the weed control spectrum but also crop safety and the mammalian and environmental safety characteristics. Biotechnology provides the opportunity to use broad-spectrum herbicides, with the desired mammalian and environmental safety characteristics,

---

[1] corresponding author

but which lack crop selectivity, and engineer selectivity into the target crop. This is the basis for the development of soybeans that are tolerant to the glyphosate, the active ingredient in the herbicide Roundup®.

Glyphosate is a non-selective, broad-spectrum, post-emergent herbicide that cannot currently be used during the growing season for soybeans or other crops, due to the sensitivity of the crop plants. Engineering glyphosate tolerance into soybeans will provide the grower with effective control of the majority of annual and perennial grasses and broad-leaved weeds in a cost effective manner. Furthermore, glyphosate has excellent environmental features, such as rapid soil binding that prevents leaching and biodegradation, which decreases persistence, as well as extremely low toxicity to mammals, birds and fish (Malik et al., 1989). Recently, glyphosate was classified by the Environmental Protection Agency as Category E (evidence of non-carcinogenicity for humans). Furthermore, Roundup® herbicide is already approved and used as both a pre-emergent and pre-harvest herbicide in soybeans. Glyphosate-tolerant soybeans would provide the grower a new broad-spectrum weed control option with an environmentally sound herbicide that works through a new mode-of-action for in-season weed control. This would allow the grower increased flexibility to treat weeds on a post-emergent basis and provides an excellent fit with reduced tillage and no tillage programs.

GTS were developed through over ten years of research. Steinrucken and Amrhein (1980) demonstrated that glyphosate acts by inhibition of 5-enolpyruvyl-shikimate-3-phosphate synthase (EPSPS), an enzyme in the aromatic amino acid biosynthetic pathway. Inhibition of EPSPS prevents synthesis of the aromatic amino acids that are essential for protein synthesis. Plants, bacteria and fungi, but not animals, contain EPSPS. Animals obtain aromatic amino acids from the food supply. Glyphosate-tolerant plants remain unaffected by glyphosate treatment, due to the presence of a glyphosate-tolerant EPSPS.

GTS have been extensively field tested over the last three years, with over 300 field tests, including approximately 200 field tests with the specific line that is being commercialized. These tests have shown GTS are tolerant to the Roundup® herbicide at a level required to control the targeted weed species. The yield of the soybean varieties containing this trait and sprayed with the Roundup® herbicide are comparable to the line not treated with the Roundup® herbicide. Data collected from these field tests have also shown that these soybeans are comparable to the parental line and other commercial varieties in morphology, outcrossing, the lack of weediness characteristics and other parameters that have been used to establish that these soybeans pose no unique environmental concerns. These data have been used to obtain the non-regulated status from the United States Department of Agriculture (USDA, 1994).

In this report, information will be summarized on the compositional and nutritional equivalence of these soybeans and the safety of the introduced protein to establish that the GTS are substantially equivalent to the soybeans currently in commerce. This information will focus on the composition of the soybeans, including analysis of selected processed soybean fractions.

Glyphosate-tolerant EPSPS

The specific glyphosate-tolerant EPSPS protein that is expressed in the glyphosate-tolerant soybeans is encoded by a gene obtained from a common soil microorganism, specifically strain *Agrobacterium* sp. CP4 (Padgette et al., 1994). Hence, the name of the protein, CP4 EPSPS. This EPSPS protein is naturally highly tolerant to glyphosate, with similar catalytic properties in the presence and absence of glyphosate. The gene and deduced amino acid sequence of the CP4 EPSPS protein have been determined. All crops and microbial food sources contain EPSPS proteins. EPSPSs present in food show a wide range of amino acid sequences. The amino acid sequence of the CP4 EPSPS shows a similar level of relatedness to the EPSPS proteins in foods as do the various EPSPS proteins in food (e.g. the CP4 EPSPS shows a comparable similarity to the EPSPS from *Bacillus subtilis*, Baker's yeast or food plants as the soybean EPSPS is to the *B. subtilis* EPSPS). Furthermore, amino acid sequences that have been shown by Monsanto to be important for EPSPS function are conserved in the CP4 EPSPS (Padgette et al., 1994). Recent studies also show that the 3-dimensional crystal structure of the CP4 EPSPS exhibits the same overall folding pattern as the *E. coli* EPSPS (D. Niedhart, W. Stallings, S. Padgette, Monsanto unpublished results).

Production of glyphosate-tolerant soybeans

Particle gun transformation was used to introduce the CP4 EPSPS gene into soybean plants (Padgette et al., 1994). A chloroplast transit peptide sequence was fused to the 5'-end of the CP4 EPSPS gene to target the CP4 EPSPS to the chloroplast, the site of aromatic amino acid synthesis and the site of the endogenous soybean EPSPS protein (della-Cioppa et al., 1986). The GTS that will be commercialized contain only a single copy of the CP4 EPSPS gene. The size and stability of this inserted gene has been well characterized using both Southern blotting and polymerase chain reaction approaches. This gene is inherited in a stable, Mendelian inheritance, as expected for a single, dominant gene. The CP4 EPSPS gene has been introduced into numerous commercial soybean varieties through traditional breeding to provide soybean growers with appropriate varieties for various soybean growing areas.

Detailed compositional and nutritional analyses were conducted on the initial GTS line 40-3-2 and the parental line to confirm that the glyphosate-tolerant soybeans, with the introduced CP4 EPSPS gene, are substantially equivalent to soybeans currently in commerce.

Compositional equivalence

The extent and specific compositional components analyzed in a food and feed assessment program should be based on the uses of the product being assessed. For soybean, the primary use is for animal feed, with approximately 97 per cent of soybean meal used for animal feed annually in the United States (Horan, 1974). The majority of the remaining 3 per cent of soybean meal is used for a variety of human food products, including bakery products, meat products, textured foods and nutritional supplements (Waggle and Kolar, 1979). Soybean oil is also the major edible oil in the United States (Mounts, 1988).

Over 1400 analytical analyses have been conducted which establish that the composition of GTS line 40-3-2 is substantially equivalent to the non-engineered, parental control variety and to other soybean varieties in commerce. These analyses have focused on both the nutrients and anti-nutrients present in soybeans. The data generated show that, in all but a few instances, for every parameter examined there was no statistically significant differences between the data for the 40-3-2 line and the parental variety. In those few instance where a difference was observed or in cases where the available data did not permit a statistical analysis, the values were well within established ranges (or fully consistent with the intended effect) as documented in the published literature.

To establish substantial equivalence, the analytical evaluation was focused on the raw agricultural product, the soybean seed. It is reasonable to infer that if the nutrient and anti-nutrient composition of the raw soybean seed for line 40-3-2 is substantial equivalent to the parental variety, then the processed products derived from 40-3-2 would also be substantially equivalent. Selected processed products (toasted meal, defatted flour, protein isolate, protein concentrate, crude lecithin and refine, bleached, deodorized oil) were produced and evaluated that confirmed this expectation.

Analysis of the important nutrients confirmed that the soybeans produced from line 40-3-2 were substantially equivalent to those produced by the parental variety and were well within the ranges published in the literature. Data obtained from seed produced at ten field locations in 1992, established that the macro-nutrients (protein, fat, fiber, ash, carbohydrate, calories and moisture) for 40-3-2 were comparable to the parental variety and published information. Likewise, there were no significant differences in the specific fatty acids or amino acids between these two lines. Particular attention was paid to the aromatic amino acids (phenylalanine, tyrosine and tryptophan) since the EPSPS protein catalyzes a reaction in the aromatic amino acid biosynthetic pathway. Since EPSPS catalyzes a non-rate-limiting step in this pathway (Herrmann, 1983), introduction of the CP4 EPSPS was not expected to alter the flux through this pathway. This was substantiated by the lack of any differences in the aromatic amino acids between GTS and the parental variety.

GTS were also shown to be substantially equivalent to the parental soybean variety in terms of the levels of specific anti-nutrients. There were no significant differences in the levels of trypsin inhibitors, lectins, phytoestrogens (genistein and daidzein), stachyose, raffinose and phytate for GTS and the parental variety. Since soybeans cannot be consumed raw by human, primarily due to the anti-nutritive activity of the trypsin inhibitors (Rackis, 1974; Rackis et al., 1986), the susceptibility of the trypsin inhibitors to inactivation upon processed was assessed. The impact of processing on lectins was also assessed as well as on urease, a standard protein that is typically used to assess the extent of processing (Herkelman et al., 1991). Levels of all three of these components were reduced to levels comparable with those reported in the literature and to levels similar for both line 40-3-2 and the parental variety. This data confirms that lines 40-30-2 and the parental control are substantially equivalent both in the levels of these anti-nutritional components in the raw agricultural products and in the inactivation of these components upon processing.

Analysis of other selected processed fractions confirmed that the composition of protein, fat, fiber, ash, carbohydrate, calories and moisture in toasted soybean meal, defatted flour, protein isolate and protein concentrate were comparable between these fractions produced from line 40-3-2 and the parental control. The fatty acid composition of refined, bleached, deodorized oil was also comparable for this processed fraction for both lines.

Finally, the composition and levels of endogenous allergens in GTS was shown to be substantially equivalent to the parental and commercial soybean varieties (Burks and Fuchs, 1994). Soybean and soybean products are well known to contain allergenic proteins (Burks et al., 1988; Maroz and Wang, 1980; Herian et al., 1990; Bush et al., 1988; Shibasaki et al., 1980). The endogenous allergenic proteins in proteins extracts from GTS were compared to the endogenous allergenic proteins from both the parental variety as well as three commercial preparations of soybean flour by the immunoblotting procedure described by Burks et al., 1988. No qualitative or quantitative differences were observed, confirming the substantial equivalence of GTS to soybeans currently in the food supply.

The extensive compositional data on the raw soybeans and processed fractions that is summarized in **Table 1** clearly establishes that GTS are substantially equivalent to the parental variety and soybeans currently in commerce.

Nutritional equivalence

Since the primary use (approximately 97 per cent) of soybeans is as a supplement for animal feed, selected animal wholesomeness studies were conducted to confirm the substantial equivalence of the soybeans derived from the glyphosate-tolerant line as compared to the parental variety. Based on the gene inserted, the method used to introduce the gene and the extensive compositional analysis performed, no differences were expected. This expectation was confirmed in wholesomeness studies performed with rat, chicken, cow, catfish and quail. There were no statistically significant differences in feed conversions in any of these wholesomeness studies between the glyphosate-tolerant soybeans and the parental variety. These studies were designed as wholesomeness studies (to measure the ability to support typical growth and well-being of the animal) and were not designed to be a toxicological studies. Such studies should be performed with particular care to assure appropriately balanced and reasonable nutritional diets (FDA, 1992; IFBC, 1990; OECD, 1993). (Refer to a paper presented at this meeting by Bruce Hammond for more detail on the design and potential concerns of these studies.) Wholesomeness studies of this type should only be carried out as a confirmatory study and only with animal species that typically consume these products as part of their diet (e.g. soybeans fed to chickens, cows, catfish, etc.).

CP4 EPSPS synthase

In addition to confirming the compositional and nutritional equivalence of GTS to commercial soybeans, the safety of the introduced CP4 EPSPS protein was also confirmed. The CP4 EPSPS is expressed very low levels in GTS, accounting for between 0.019 and 0.040 per cent of the soybean seed by weight, as determined with validated ELISA assays with seed derived from ten field tests conducted in 1992. CP4 EPSPS accounted for no more than 0.1 per cent of the total protein in either soybean seed or processed fractions prepared from these soybeans. As expected, CP4 EPSPS activity was not detected in toasted soybean meal fractions, protein isolate or protein concentrate prepared from these soybeans due to inactivation upon processing.

Based on the reaction catalyzed, CP4 EPSPS is functionally similar to the EPSPS proteins typically present in food and feed derived from plant and microbial sources. The structural relationship between CP4 EPSPS and other food EPSPSs is demonstrated by the amino acid sequence comparison, the homology of active sites residues and the three-dimensional structure.

To confirm the mammalian safety of the CP4 EPSPS protein, the CP4 EPSPS was shown to be rapidly degraded in a simulated mammalian digestion experiment, to show no adverse treated related effects in an acute mouse gavage study, to show no significant amino acid homology to known protein toxins or allergens and to pose no significant allergenic concerns. For these experiments, the CP4 EPSPS protein was produced in *E. coli* (Padgette et al., 1994). This protein was demonstrated to be equivalent to the CP4 EPSPS purified from the seed of the glyphosate-tolerance soybeans. The CP4 EPSPS protein was shown to be rapidly degraded in both the simulated gastric and intestinal systems. No treatment related adverse effects were observed in administering the purified CP4 EPSPS protein at over a thousand-fold safety factor to mice in an acute gavage study. Acute administration was used to assess the safety of the CP4 EPSPS since proteins that are toxic act via acute mechanisms (Sjoblad et al., 1992; Pariza and Foster, 1983; Jones and Maryanski, 1991). Finally, the deduced amino acid sequence of the CP4 EPSPS was shown to have no significant homology to the known protein toxins or allergens in the three established data basis (Pearson and Lipman, 1988; Wilbur and Lipman, 1983; Pearson, 1990; Gribskov and Devereux, 1992).

The CP4 EPSPS protein was shown to pose no significant allergenic concerns by comparing the biochemical properties of the CP4 EPSPS to the properties of commonly allergenic proteins (Padgette et al., 1994). Whereas commonly allergenic proteins are typically between 10,000 and 70,000 daltons in size, prevalent in food, stable to the acidic and proteolytic conditions of the digestive system, stable to food processing and glycosylated (**Table 2**), the CP4 EPSPS protein shares only a similar molecular weight, but none of the other characteristics. Furthermore, CP4 EPSPS shares no significant amino acid homology to known allergens. Although none of these biochemical criteria alone enable prediction of the allergenic potential of proteins, the combination of these characteristics provide a strong bases to conclude that the CP4 EPSPS poses no significant allergenic concerns.

The safety of the CP4 EPSPS has been confirmed by demonstrating the rapid degradation of this protein in simulated digestive system, performing an acute mouse gavage study and assessing its allergenic potential.

Glyphosate-tolerant soybeans are substantially equivalent to soybeans in commerce

The extensive compositional and nutritional analysis performed clearly establish that the insertion of the CP4 EPSPS gene and expression of the CP4 EPSPS protein in these soybeans to confer tolerance to glyphosate has not altered these soybeans in any significant way. These GTS are substantially equivalent to the parental soybean variety and to soybeans currently in commerce.

Table 1
Summary of the Compositional Analyses Performed on Glyphosate-tolerant Soybean Products

Component	Raw beans	Toasted meal
Proximate analysis[2]	SE	SE
Amino acid	SE	NA
Fatty acid	SE	NA
Trypsin inhibitors	SE	SE
Lectins	SE	SE
Phytoestrogens	SE	SE
Urease	SE	SE
Stachyose, raffinose	NA	SE
Phytate	NA	SE

SE = substantially equivalent to the control
NA = not analyzed
[2] = Typically but not absolutely

Table 2
Comparison of the Biochemical Characteristics of CP4 EPSPS and Known Allergenic Proteins[1]

Characteristic	Allergens	CP4 EPSPS
Molecular wt. 10-70 kd	yes	yes
Prevalent protein in food	yes	no
Stable to digestion	yes	no
Stable to processing	yes	no
Glycosylated	yes[2]	no
Similar to known allergens	—[3]	no
Similar to soybean proteins	—	yes

[1] As described by Taylor (1992) and Taylor et al. (1987, 1992)
[2] Typically but not absolutely
[3] Implicit for allergenic proteins from soybeans

Application of the principles of substantial equivalence to other genetically-engineered plant products

The detailed approaches used to establish that GTS are substantially equivalent to current varieties of soybeans has also been applied to several other genetically-engineered products that we are planning to market. These examples confirm the value and applicability of the substantial equivalence approach to assess the safety of genetically-engineered plant products and confirms that many of these products are substantially equivalent to current commercial products. Assessments similar to that described for glyphosate-tolerant soybeans have been completed for the following products: cotton resistant to lepidopteran insect pests, potato resistant to the Colorado potato beetle, canola tolerant to glyphosate, tomato with delayed ripening and cotton tolerant to glyphosate. Extremely low levels of the proteins encoded by the introduced genes are expressed in these products. These proteins are all rapidly degraded in simulated digestion studies and have been shown to cause no adverse effects in acute mouse gavage studies at levels exceeding one-thousand fold higher than the maximal anticipated consumption levels.

Analyses of over 450 different nutritional or anti-nutritional components for 20 lines for these six different crops (including GTS) have confirmed that each of these genetically-engineered products are substantially equivalent to the non-engineered varieties used today. Furthermore, appropriate animal wholesomeness studies with each of these products have also confirmed that there are not meaningful nutritional differences between these products and the products currently in the market.

These collective data totally support the approach of substantial equivalence that has been recommended by OECD (1993) and the FDA Food Policy (1992) in assessing the safety of genetically-engineered plant products.

References

Burks, A.W., Brooks, J.R. and Sampson, H.A. (1988) Allergenicity of major component proteins of soybean determined by enzyme linked immunosorbent assay (ELISA) and immunoblotting in children with atopic dermatitis and positive soy challenges. *J. Allergy Clin. Immunol.* 81:1135-11423.

Burks, A.W. and Fuchs, R.L. (1994) Assessment of the endogenous allergens in glyphosate-tolerant and commercial soybean varieties. *J. Allergy Clin. Immunol.* (in press)

Bush, R.K., Schroeckenstein, D., Meier-Davis, S., Balmes, J. and D. Rempel (1988) Soybean flour asthma: detection of allergens by immunoblotting. *J. Allergy Clin. Immunol.* 82:251-255.

della-Cioppa, G., Bauer, S.C., Klein, B.K. Shah, D.M., Fraley, R.T. and Kishore, G. (1986) Translocation of the precursor of 5-enolpyruvylshikimate-3-phosphate synthase into chloroplasts of higher plants *in vitro*. *Proc. Natl. Acad. Sci.* USA 83:6873-6877.

Gianessi, L.P. and Puffer, C. (1991) *Herbicide use in the United States.* Resources for the Future, Washington, D.C.

Gribskov, M. and Devereux, J. (1992) *Sequence Analysis Primer*. W. H. Freeman and Co., New York.

Herian, A.M., Taylor, S.L. and Robert, K.B. (1990) Identification of soybean allergens by immunoblotting with sera from soy-allergic adults. *Int. J. Allergy Appl. Immunol.* 92:193-198.

Herkelman, K.L., Cromwell, G.L. and Stahly, T.S. (1991) Effects of heating time and sodium metabisulfite on the nutritional value of full-fat soybeans for chicks. *J. Animal Sci.* 69:4477-4486.

Herrmann, K.M. (1983) The Common Aromatic Biosynthetic Pathway. In: *Amino Acids: Biosynthesis and Genetic Regulation* (K.M. Kerrmann and R.L. Somerville, eds.) Addison-Wesley, Reading, Massachusets, 301-322.

Horan, F.E. (1974) Soy protein products and their production. *J. Am. Oil Chemists' Soc.* 51:67A-73A.

International Food Biotechnology Council (1990) Biotechnologies and food: assuring the safety of food produced by genetic modification. *Regulatory Toxicol. Pharmacol.* 12:S1-S196.

Jones, D.D. and Maryanski, J.H. (1991) Safety Considerations in the Evaluation of Transgenic Plants for Human Foods. In: *Risk Assessment in Genetic Engineering* (M.A. Levin and H.S. Strauss, eds.). McGraw-Hill, New York, 64-82.

Malik, J., Barry, G. and Kishore, G. (1989) The herbicide glyphosate. *BioFactors* 2:17-25.

Maroz, L.A. and Wang, W.H. (1980) Kunitz soybean trypsin-inhibitor: a specific allergen in food anaphylaxis. *N. Engl. J. Med.* 302:1126-1128.

Mounts, T.L. (1988) Edible Soybean Oil Products. In: *Soybean Utilization Alternatives* (L. McCann, ed.) Center for Alternative Crops and Products, Univ. Minn., St. Paul, Minnesota, 43-56.

OECD (1993) *Safety Evaluation of Foods Derived by Modern Biotechnology: Concepts and Principles*. Paris.

Padgette, S.R., Re, D.B., Barry, G.F., Eichholtz, D.A., Delannay, X., Fuchs, R.L., Kishore, G.M. and Fraley, R.T. (1994) *New Weed Control Opportunities: Development of Soybeans with Roundup® tolerance*. In: Herbicide-Resistant Crops: Agricultural Economic, Environmental, Regulatory, and Technological Aspects (S.O. Duke, ed.). CRC Press. (in press)

Pariza, M.W. and Foster, E.M. (1983) Determining the safety of enzymes used in food processing. *J. Food Protection* 46:453-468.

Pearson, W. and Lipman, D. (1988) Improved tools for biological sequence comparison. PNAS USA 85:2444-2448.

Pearson, W.R. (1990) Rapid and sensitive sequence comparison with FASTP and FASTA. *Methods Enzymol.* 183:63-98.

Rackis, J.J. (1974) Biological and physiological factors in soybeans. *J. Am. Oil Chemists' Soc.* 51:161A-173A.

Rackis, J.J., Wolf, W.J. and Baker, E.C. (1986) Protease Inhibitors in Plant Foods: Content and Inactivation. In: *Nutritional and Toxicological Significance of Enzyme Inhibitors in Food.* (M. Friedman, ed.) Plenum Press, New York, 299-347.

Shibasaki, M., Suzuki, S., Tajima, S., Nemoto, H. and Kuroume, T. (1980) Allergenicity of major component proteins in soybean. *Int. Arch. Allergy Appl. Immunol.* 61:441-448.

Sjoblad, R.D., McClintock, J.T. and Engler, R. (1992) Toxicological considerations for protein components of biological pesticide products. *Regulatory Toxicol. and Pharmacol.* 15:3-9.

Steinrucken, H.C. and Amrhein, N. (1980) The herbicide glyphosate is a potent inhibitor of 5-enolpyruvyl shikimic acid-3-phosphate synthase. *Biochem. Biophys. Res. Com.* 94:1207-1212.

Taylor, S.L. (1992) Chemistry and detection of food allergens. *Food Technol.* 39:146-152.

Taylor, S.L., Lemanske, R.F. Jr., Bush, R.K. and Busse, W.W. (1987) Food allergens: structure and immunologic properties. *Ann. Allergy* 59:93-99.

Taylor, S.L., Nordlee, J.A. and Bush, R.K. (1992) Food Allergies. In: *Food Safety Assessment*, ACS Symposium Series 484 (J.W. Finley, S.F. Robinson and D.J. Armstrong, eds.). American Chemical Society, Washington, D.C.

United States Department of Agriculturae (1994) Response to Monsanto Petition P93-258-01 for determination of nonregulated status for glyphosate tolerant soybean line 40-3-2. *Federal Register* 59:26781.

United States Food and Drug Administration (1992) Foods derived from new plant varieties. *Federal Register* 57:22984-23005.

Waggle, D.H. and Kolar, C.W. (1979) Types of Soy Protein Products. In: *Soy Protein and Human Nutrition* (H.L. Wilke, D.T. Hopkins and D.H. Waggle, eds.). Academic Press, New York, 19-51.

Wilbur, W. J. and Lipman, D. J. (1983) Improved tools for biological sequence comparison. *PNAS USA* 80:726-730.

Food Safety Evaluation of a Transgenic Squash

Hector Quemada

**Asgrow Seed Company/Upjohn
United States**

The food will be talking about this afternoon will be different from the foods that have been discussed previously today, in that it is producing no new proteins relative to those which are produced in counterparts of the food presently being consumed. For this reason we can consider this food not to be novel, even though the process used to produce it might have been. Therefore, this food can be regarded as being substantially equivalent, and even virtually identical, to food on the market today.

As a framework for this discussion, I will be using the decision tree published by the US Food and Drug Administration in their Statement of Policy published in 1992. While these decision trees did not dictate the direction of our food safety work, much of the information which has been generated during the development of this genetically modified variety, as well as other varieties produced via traditional plant breeding, can be used to answer the questions asked in the decision trees.

As the US FDA rightly points out in its Statement of Policy, much information which is useful for the assessment of safety is contained in the base of knowledge which breeders accumulate during their work. Consequently, safety assessments can make use of the existing base of information, which includes the published literature as well as knowledge of standard agricultural practices and characteristics of the particular crop being considered. In assessing the food safety of transgenic squash, we have attempted to adhere as closely as possible to standard practices used to assess the safety of other traditionally bred varieties of squash.

The transgenic squash line ZW20 has been engineered to be resistant to two viruses – zucchini yellow mosaic virus (ZYMV) and watermelon mosaic virus 2 (WMV2) – which are serious pathogens of this and other cucurbit crops worldwide. When non-transgenic, virus-susceptible plants are infected with the ZYMV and WMV2, plants develop distorted leaves and are stunted. The fruit are distorted and discolored, causing them to be unmarketable.

In order to introduce virus resistance into this crop, the coat proteins of the viruses have been cloned, and engineered for expression by attachment of the cauliflower mosaic virus 35S promoter and polyadenylation sequences. The squash was transformed using *Agrobacterium tumefaciens* to transfer the coat protein genes via a binary plasmid vector.

I will now proceed through the FDA decision trees and discuss the reasons which justify our answers to the questions asked.

Does the host species have a history of safe use?

Yes. The particular species of squash in question is *Cucurbita pepo* L. The fact that the name "squash" is derived from a northeastern Native American word (Whitaker and Robinson, 1986) is indicative of its historical use as a food. Evidence of use in pre-Colombian times has been obtained from archaeological sites, indicating domestication of *C. pepo* dating to perhaps 7000 years ago (Smith, 1992) and more clearly by 3000 years ago (Heiser, 1989; Smith, 1992). The large number of varieties of *C. pepo* make it a vegetable which is consumed worldwide.

The specific variety of *C. pepo* in question is a yellow crookneck type, classified as *Cucurbita pepo* subsp. *ovifera* (L.) Decker var. *ovifera* (Decker, 1988). The yellow crookneck squash type is consumed throughout the United States, but primarily in the Southeast. It is consumed mostly as a fresh vegetable, eaten either cooked or raw. The specific line of squash which has served as the host plant for the genetic modification is the yellow crookneck line YC77E. It has been used as a parent for a commercial yellow crookneck hybrid sold by Asgrow Seed Company for eight years.

Do characteristics of the host species, related species, or progenitor lines warrant analytical or toxicological tests?

No. Cucurbits, including squash, are known to produce very bitter alkaloids known as cucurbitacins. Two genes are known to control production of these alkaloids: *Bi*, a dominant gene which controls the production of high cucurbitacin content; and *cu*, a recessive gene which directs the synthesis of reduced levels of cucurbitacin B (Whitaker and Robinson, 1986). Elevated levels of cucurbitacins are readily detectable by taste. In fact, the sense of taste is known to be extremely sensitive to cucurbitacin, with documented sensitivity as low as 1 part per billion for cucurbitacin B and 10 ppb for cucurbitacin E glycoside (Metcalf et al., 1980; Rymal et al., 1984). The latter is the primary cucurbitacin in squash (Rehm et al., 1957). The detection levels by taste are 34,000 times lower than the reported oral LD_{50} in mice (Merck Index, 1989). Cucurbitacin E is the only cucurbitacin documented to have caused harm in normal human diets; breeding and isolation during production are standard methods of reducing risk (Coulston and Kolbye, 1990).

Because of the extreme bitterness of cucurbitacin E, a standard test for the presence of this compound in squash breeding programmes involves the tasting of fruits to determine bitterness. Breeders pay special attention to the elimination of bitterness especially, when undomesticated relatives are used in the parentage leading to a commercial product. Lines with bitterness are eliminated from development. The unmodified yellow crookneck squash line is itself non-bitter and the transgenic line, ZW20, is non-bitter as well. Therefore, since elevated levels of cucurbitacin have not been detected, toxicological tests are not warranted.

Table 1
Compositional Analysis of Transgenic Squash, Corresponding Commercial Variety, and Values in the Literature

Component	Transgenic	Non-transgenic	Literature (Pennington, 1989)
Protein (g/100g)	0.8-1.2	0.8-1.4	0.9
Moisture (g/100g)	93.6-94.5	93.7-94.8	94.2
Fat (g/100g)	<0.1-0.1	<0.1	0.3
Ash (g/100g)	0.4-0.7	0.5-0.8	
Total dietary fiber (g/100g)	1.0-1.2	1.0-1.1	1.1
Carbohydrates (g/100g)	4.1-4.3	3.9-4.4	4.0
Calories (Calories/100g)	16.4-18.9	14.4-18.4	18.5
Fructose (g/100g)	0.9-1.2	1.1-1.3	
Glucose (g/100g)	0.8-1.1	1.0-1.2	
Sucrose (g/100g)	<0.2	<0.2-0.2	
Lactose (g/100g)	<0.2	<0.2	
Maltose (g/100g)	<0.2	<0.2	
Vitamin C (mg/100g)	15.1-22.4	14.1-23.2	7.7
Beta carotene (mg/100g)	<0.03-0.05	<0.03-0.04	
Vitamin A (IU/100g)	<50-80	<50-70	338
Calcium (mg/100g)	13.3-29.4	15.7-29.7	21.5
Iron (mg/100g)	0.287-0.367	0.372-0.478	0.477
Sodium (mg/100g)	<2.50-3.98	<2.50-2.86	

Is the concentration and bioavailability of important nutrients in the new variety within the range ordinarily seen in the host species?

Yes. The compositional analysis of squash plants grown in three separate field locations under typical agricultural conditions revealed that the concentrations of nutrients in transformed squash compared with the non-transgenic counterpart or published values were typical for this crop. The compositional analysis is given in **Table 1**. The single measurement which varies significantly from the published literature is the amount of vitamin A. However, this value is the same in the non-transgenic as in the transgenic fruit, and cannot be attributed to the transformation process. This difference can readily be accounted for by differences between the harvest times of the fruit used as the basis for the literature values and the fruit used in the present analysis.

Safety Assessment of new varieties: the donors

Table 1 presents the compositional analysis of transgenic squash, the corresponding commercial variety, and values in the literature. The commercial variety is produced as an F1 hybrid, with one of the parents being the line subsequently used for genetic transformation. The transgenic variety is also a hybrid, made of the same parental lines, but with the transgenic version of one parent.

Is food from the donor commonly allergenic?

No. The donor organisms are zucchini yellow mosaic virus (ZYMV) and watermelon mosaic virus 2 (WMV2). These viruses are not themselves used as food, but can be found in cucurbit fruit – including squash fruit – consumed as food (Provvidenti et al., 1984). It is almost certain that food containing these and other viruses has been eaten throughout the history of human consumption of squash. None of the proteins produced by ZYMV and WMV2 is known to be an allergen. The introduced proteins, the coat proteins of these viruses, will be addressed specifically below.

Do characteristics of the donor species, related species, or progenitor lines warrant toxicological tests?

No. As stated above, the donor organisms (ZYMV and WMV2), as well as other related plant viruses, are found in cucurbits consumed as food by humans. No toxicity has been reported for these viruses. Consequently, no toxicity can be attributed to the specific proteins introduced, namely the ZYMV and WMV2 coat proteins. The coat proteins are the only portion of the ZYMV and WMV2 genomes which could have been introduced into plants, because the cloning and engineering process isolated only these genes.

The ZYMV and WMV2 coat protein genes are only genes which are contained in the ZW20 line which will be commercialized. The original transformed plant contained the gene for neomycin phosphotransferase 2 (NPT2). However, detailed molecular characterization of the T-DNA insertions in ZW20 has shown that only one intact NPT2 gene was present in the original transformant, and that this NPT2 gene was unlinked to other insertion events which contained only viral coat protein genes. Apparently, these events were the result of incomplete transfer of the T-DNA. The NPT2 gene was subsequently eliminated by Mendelian segregation. Absence of the NPT2 gene in advanced generations has been confirmed by Southern Blot analysis.

Southern Blots have also been done to determine the presence of any non-T-DNA sequences which might have been donated by the binary Ti-plasmid system derived from *Agrobacterium tumefaciens*. These tests have shown the absence of any non-T-DNA sequences.

This analysis leads to a conclusion of No Concerns for the donor organisms.

Safety assessment of new varieties: proteins introduced from donors

Is the newly introduced protein present in food derived from the plant?

Yes. The coat proteins of ZYMV and WMV2 produced under the direction of these genes are detectable at low levels in squash fruit. These fruit are used as food.

Is the protein derived from a food source, or similar to an edible protein?

Yes. The coat proteins introduced into squash are known at the amino acid sequence level. The protein produced by the expression of the engineered WMV2 gene should consist of a fusion between the WMV2 coat protein and the NH_3-terminal 16 amino acids of the CMV coat protein gene. The expression of the engineered ZYMV gene should produce a full-length ZYMV coat protein, with an added methionine residue. All coat proteins or coat protein fragments are found in abundance in squash fruit presently consumed by humans. The sequences as engineered are no more different from the original sequence than are two different strains of the same potyvirus. For example, a WMV2 strain previously identified as the N strain of soybean mosaic virus (Yu et al., 1989; Frenkel et al., 1989) possesses a coat protein which differs from that of other WMV2 strains by the absence of a stretch of 16 amino acids; these other strains in turn may differ by as much as 5 per cent in amino acid sequence (Quemada et al., 1990). The structure of these proteins is well within the range of sequence variation of viral coat proteins.

Furthermore, measurements conducted on the levels of the ZYMV, WMV2 and other viral coat proteins in market yellow crookneck squash, as well as zucchini squash, cantaloupe and honeydew melon, show that amounts of coat protein can be up to 268 times greater for ZYMV and 421 times greater for WMV2 in these foods than in ZW20 squash fruit. This is shown in **Table 2**.

Table 2
Measurements of Viral Coat Proteins in Supermarket Fruit

As measured by ELISA assay. CMV = cucumber mosaic virus coat protein; PRV = papaya ringspot virus coat protein; ZYMV = zucchini yellow mosaic virus coat protein; WMV2 = watermelon mosaic virus coat protein; ND = not detected; C1-7 are cantaloupe, H1-16 are honeydew melon, Y1-4 are yellow crookneck squash, and Z1-8 are zucchini squash. The top line is the transgenic line of squash being developed for market.

Fruit	CMV (µg/kg fruit)	PRV (µg/kg fruit)	ZYMV (µg/kg fruit)	WMV2 (µg/kg fruit)
YC77EZW20	ND	ND	68.4	430.6
C1	355,200	18,000	14,400	10,320
C2	130,464	5,472	10,944	115,488
C3	ND	252,000	28,800	720
C4	ND	ND	864	ND
C5	>2,400,000	1,200	8,400	ND
C6	>3,216,000	ND	14,000	ND
C7	>3,216,000	ND	12,864	ND
H1	ND	7,200	9,480	ND
H2	ND	6,840	1,800	ND
H3	ND	ND	2,200	ND
H4	359	4,752	3,888	173
H5	269	3,168	3,168	260
H6	238	ND	2,592	ND
H7	ND	5,928	1,824	137
H8	664	13,272	1,896	190
H9	82	960	24	24
H10	ND	ND	250	ND
H11	ND	ND	1,560	ND
H12	ND	ND	480	ND
H13	ND	ND	2,200	ND
H14	ND	3,120	720	ND
H15	ND	10,080	1,700	ND
H16	ND	ND	3,100	ND
Y1	ND	ND	11,424	ND
Y2	ND	ND	ND	ND
Y3	ND	ND	1,152	ND
Y4	ND	ND	13,056	ND
Z1	ND	ND	140	ND
Z2	ND	ND	ND	ND
Z3	ND	ND	454	ND
Z4	ND	ND	ND	ND
Z5	ND	ND	ND	ND
Z6	ND	ND	576	ND
Z7	43	ND	2,592	ND
Z8	14	ND	2,900	ND

These data are consistent with other studies (Provvidenti et al., 1994) reporting recovery of viruses, including ZYMV and WMV2, from produce collected from market samples.

Even if the answer to this question were "no", the answer to the subsequent question, "Does the biological function of the introduced protein raise any safety concern, or is the introduced protein reported to be toxic?" would be "no" because the biological function of the proteins is known and this function does not raise any safety concern. Furthermore, despite the high levels of viral coat protein in cucurbit fruit, cucurbits have historically been consumed without reports of toxicity due to coat proteins.

Is food from the donor commonly allergenic?

No. Despite the high levels of viral coat protein found in squash, viral coat proteins have not been reported to be allergenic. Plant viruses are not among the organisms commonly known to be allergenic.

Is the introduced protein reported to be toxic?

No. Despite the high levels of viral coat protein found in squash, viral coat proteins have not been reported to be toxic.

Will the intake of the donor protein in a new variety be generally comparable to the intake of the same or similar protein in donor or other food?

Yes. Measurements of ZYMV and WMV2 coat proteins show that the levels of these coat proteins in transgenic squash are within the range of coat proteins measured in market squash. The levels expressed by the introduced genes are in the lower end of the distribution of coat protein concentrations measured.

Is the introduced protein likely to be a macroconstituent in human or animal diet?

No. While large amounts of viral coat protein may be found in cucurbits consumed as a part of the human diet, the levels of viral coat protein synthesized under the direction of the introduced genes are low and will not be a macroconstituent in the human or animal diet. The concentrations of viral coat protein are in the range micrograms/kilogram of fruit, while total protein in squash, as Table 1 shows, is in the range of 10 grams/kilogram of fruit.

This analysis leads to a conclusion of No Concerns for the proteins introduced from the donors.

The safety assessment that has been conducted on this specific transgenic squash has demonstrated that it is substantially equivalent to squash presently being consumed by humans. Because we have demonstrated this, it is our conclusion that this food can be consumed with the same degree of safety as other squash varieties being sold today.

Even if the answer to this question were "no", the answer to the subsequent question, "Does the biological function of the introduced protein raise any safety concern, or is the introduced protein reported to be toxic?" would be "no", as indicated earlier.

References

Coulston, F. and Kolbye, A.C. (eds.) Biotechnologies and food: assuring the safety of foods produced by genetic modification. *Reg. Tox. Pharm.* 12:S1-S196.

Decker, D.S. (1988) Origin(s), evolution, and systematics of *Cucurbita pepo* (Cucurbitaceae). *Econ. Bot.* 42:4-15.

Frenkel, M.J., Ward, C.W. and Shukla, D.D. (1989) The use of 3' non-coding nucleotide sequences in the taxonomy of potyviruses: application to watermelon mosaic virus 2 and soybean mosaic virus-N. *J. Gen. Virol.* 70:2775-2783.

Heiser, C.B., Jr. (1989) Domestication of the Cucurbitaceae: Cucurbita and Lagenaria. In: *Foraging and Farming* (D. Harris and G. Hillman, eds.). Unwin Hyman, London.

Metcalf, R.L., Metcalf, R.A. and Rhodes, A.M. (1980) Cucurbitacins as kairomones for diabroticite beetles. *Proc. Nat. Acad. Sci.* USA 77:3769-3772.

Merck Index, 11th edition (1989). Merck and Co., Inc., Rahway, New Jersey.

Pennington, J.A.T. (1989) *Food Values of Portions Commonly Used*, 15th edition. J.B. Lippincott, Philadelphia, Pennsylvania.

Provvidenti, R., Gonsalves, D. and Humaydan, H.S. (1984) Occurrence of zucchini yellow mosaic virus in cucurbits from Connecticut, New York, Florida, and California. *Plant Disease* 68:443-446.

Quemada, H., Sieu, L.C., Siemieniak, D.R., Gonsalves, D. and Slightom, J.L. (1990) Watermelon mosaic virus II and zucchini yellow mosaic virus: cloning of 3'-terminal regions, nucleotide sequences, and phylogenetic comparisons. *J. Gen. Virol.* 71:1451-1460.

Rehm, S., Enslin, P.R., Meeuse, A.D.J. and Wessels, J.H. (1957) Bitter principles of the Cucurbitaceae. VII. The distribution of bitter principles in this plant family. *J. Sci. Food Agr.* 8:679-686.

Rymal, K.S., Chambliss, O.L., Bond, M.D. and Smith, D.A. (1984) Squash containing toxic cucurbitacin compounds occurring in California and Alabama. *Journal of Food Protection* 47:270-271.

Smith, B.D. (1992) Rivers of Change – Essays on Early Agriculture in Eastern North America. Smithsonian Institution Press, Washington, D.C.

Whitaker, T.W. and R.W. Robinson (1986) Squash breeding. In: *Breeding Vegetable Crops* (Mark J. Basset, ed.). Avi Publishing Company, Inc., Westport, Connecticut.

Yu, M.H., Frenkel, M.J., McKern, N.M., Shukla, D.D., Strike, P.M. and Ward, C.W. (1989) Coat protein of potyviruses. 6. Amino acid sequences suggest watermelon mosaic virus 2 and soybean mosaic virus-N are strains of the same potyvirus. *Arch. Virol.* 105:55-64.

Evaluation of Strategies for Food Safety Assessment of Genetically Modified Agricultural Products – Information Needs

E.J. Kok and H.A. Kuiper

State Institute for Quality Control of Agricultural Products
The Netherlands

Introduction

The use of gene technology in food production has enabled microbiologists, and animal and plant breeders, to establish genetic combinations that could not be obtained by means of classical breeding procedures. Thereby it has proved feasible to add or improve specific (qualitative) characteristics in microbial, plant and animal species. Novel foods, when related to genetic modification, may either contain food ingredients produced by genetically modified organisms, or consist of or contain such organisms.

Because of these scientific developments, national and international regulatory bodies have considered the question of how adequate existing regulation is with respect to food safety aspects of novel foods derived from genetically modified organisms. This has resulted in a number of advisory reports proposing different strategies for risk assessment. In the proposal for a European Parliament and Council regulation[1] these issues are summarized as:

1) The products should be safe for the consumer when consumed at the intended level of use.

2) The products should not mislead the consumer.

3) The products should not differ from similar food or food ingredients that they may replace in the diet in such a way that their normal consumption would be nutritionally disadvantageous for the consumer.

In this paper the differences between proposed risk assessment strategies are briefly discussed, as well as ways to improve such strategies in the future.

Food safety

Many organisms, microorganisms, plants and animals have a long history of use as foods. These organisms have been bred and selected to improve specific characteristics. "Selection might have included an evaluation of safety, although it was not formally recognized. In any case, there is little historical record or documentation of the process by which the safety of food plants was maintained..."[2] Traditional foods are considered safe, although it is now generally recognized that some of these products contain substances that may be harmful to the consumer when consumed in significant quantities. Fundamental knowledge about the biochemical background of selection traits, for example disease resistance, is often lacking. In the Netherlands and most other countries, no specific product regulation exists with respect to new food products of plant or animal origin. The only substances determined on a regular basis are glycoalkaloids in new potato varieties and nitrate in leaf vegetables.

The production of novel foods derived from genetically modified organisms has stimulated regulatory authorities to consider the necessity of additional regulation for this new type of products. Reports on the subject have been published by:

- International Food Biotechnology Council (1990)

- Scandinavia: Nordic Working Group on Food Toxicology and Risk Assessment (1991)

- United Kingdom: Advisory Committee on Novel Foods and Processes (1991)

- FAO/WHO (1991)

- Netherlands: Health Council and Food Council (1992/1993)

- United States: Food and Drug Administration (1992)

- OECD (1993)

In preparation:

- EU: DG III

A report evaluating the different food safety assessment strategies described in these advisory reports was published in 1993.[3]

The proposed guidelines for evaluating the safety aspects of novel foods show great similarity with respect to the basic elements of the safety evaluation: toxicity, exposure and the OECD-formulated principle of substantial equivalence. Differences can be seen with respect to the necessity for additional tests to determine, for example, toxicity and allergenicity. One discussion point is whether feeding trials with the complex product should be part of the standard toxicological risk evaluation. In view of the problems encountered with animal experiments when complex food products are involved (difficulties in composing a balanced diet, low safety factors), the choice of a more analytical approach seems to be justified. Most reports advocate a combined toxicological and analytical approach providing a more detailed molecular and physiological basis for risk assessment procedures. Such procedures usually include nutritional aspects as well.

The case-by-case approach is generally accepted as the best one for evaluating the great variety of novel food products that are moving towards the market. Nevertheless, there is considerable variation in the room for manoeuvre between the different approaches. Some proposals for risk evaluation are based on dividing new products into different categories (especially the IFBC and the Dutch advisory organs), whereas the OECD applies the case-by-case approach in the most far-reaching way. In this sense, the more recent proposals tend more towards the case-by-case approach.

In a number of countries, specific regulations for novel food products are currently being implemented. The approval of novel foods for the market in the Netherlands is a two-step procedure. Firstly, food safety is assessed by the Provisional Committee on the Safety of Novel Foods; secondly, other aspects of the food product, for example labelling, are considered in the Novel Foods Committee. In general, it can be stated that in those countries that have adopted a novel foods regulation, new food products derived from genetically modified organisms are extensively assessed. The testing requirements, however, may differ from country to country and in general the testing methods can be improved.

As the room for manoeuvre of most (proposed) guidelines is quite considerable, it is not clear to what extent the introduction of these guidelines will result in conformity of evaluations of new products in the different countries. It is anticipated that the risk evaluation of single substances and simple chemical mixtures will usually not show major differences in the different countries. Also, in relation to the evaluation of genetically modified microorganisms, no major contrasts can be observed in the different proposals. It can be seen, however, that when introducing evaluation strategies for transgenic plant and animal products, there will be major differences in the risk evaluations. The OECD and other international organisations, in particular, advocate evaluation based on molecular and biochemical analysis, comparing the new product with its traditional counterpart. The FDA also advises novel food producers to follow the analytical approach. The Scandinavian and Dutch reports, on the other hand, tend to base the evaluation on toxicity tests of the product. It would therefore be valuable to make an evaluation of approved products and of the criteria that have been applied in order to develop an internationally accepted evaluation strategy. It is obvious that international harmonization of the safety requirements for novel foods will be necessary to avoid new trade traffic barriers, and it is therefore important that international organisations such as the OECD take the lead in the discussion on guidelines for novel foods and novel food ingredients derived from genetically modified organisms.

At this moment, a few bottlenecks can be identified with respect to the improvement of risk assessment strategies. It will first be necessary to develop new toxicological concepts when assessing complex novel foods. Classical toxicological concepts, such as animal feeding trials, have been developed for single substances such as drugs or food additives. As stated earlier, when applying those methods to complex products derived from genetically modified food organisms a number of problems are met that can not easily be resolved. In classical animal feeding trials with complex food products, it will usually not be possible to combine a balanced diet with safety factors that are in general required in this type of study. Moreover, such trials may result in data that are difficult to interpret. New toxicological concepts should therefore not be based solely on classical toxicity testing, but combine analytical methods with (newly developed) *in vitro* systems and traditional toxicology. Analytical methods may be based on information at DNA, mRNA or metabolic level.

At this moment, the information on changes at the DNA level can be informative but will usually not be sufficient to assess possible changes in the physiology of the organism. Additional mRNA or metabolite profiles may help overcome this problem. Metabolite profiling refers to the determination of potential differences in the composition of macronutrients, micronutrients and natural toxins in genetically modified products and their traditional counterpart by means of a number of analytical and chemical techniques, such as infrared spectroscopy, nuclear magnetic resonance spectroscopy, gas chromatography, mass spectrometry and high-performance liquid chromatography. If there are any indications for changes in the metabolism of the organism, *in vitro* systems can be very helpful in further identifying the significance of such changes. Only the fraction of the organism that showed any changes in its metabolite profile needs to be further investigated in *in vitro* systems, in those cases where analysis of the fraction does not supply sufficient information on the toxicological relevance of the altered composition. In this concept the necessity for subacute or semichronic toxicity studies needs to be shown prior to their performance, whereas nowadays these studies are often carried out without the possibility to predict their relevance.

When discussing analytical methods as part of a risk assessment procedure for novel foods, we encounter a second bottleneck. In order to be able to identify possible significant (toxicological) changes, we need to know what natural compositional variation occurs in (varieties of) the specific organism. In general, current data systems on the composition of traditional foods cannot supply detailed information on, for example, variation in the presence of natural toxins or specific macro-/micronutrients in various tissues in different varieties of food species. We need new data systems that gather existing data in this field, supplemented with data from specific research projects.

Another bottleneck in risk assessment procedures relates to immunotoxicity testing, in particular allergenicity testing. Immunotoxicity is a relatively new field in experimental research. In general, a protein or a protein fragment can cause an immunological effect when a certain epitope is introduced unchanged or when the protein, or fragment, has been modified in such a way that an effect can occur. At this moment, however, there is no method available to screen new food proteins on allergenicity. And as basic immunotoxicological knowledge is limited, the development of such methods cannot be foreseen in the near future. Major research efforts will be necessary to fill this knowledge gap.

Conclusions

The number of novel food products derived from genetically modified complex food organisms is increasing. As a result, national and international regulatory bodies are considering the necessity for additional regulations to ensure the food safety of these novel foods. In the last few years, several advisory reports have been published on the subject and it can be concluded that the key elements in the different proposed strategies to evaluate the safety of novel foods are largely the classical toxicological elements, toxicity and exposure, supplemented by "the OECD component", substantial equivalence. Differences can be seen with respect to the necessity for additional testing of (immuno)toxicity by means of animal feeding trials. Criteria for approval of a new product are far from clear. To gain more insight into these criteria, and to work towards an internationally accepted evaluation strategy, it would be valuable to make an evaluation of approved products and of the criteria that have been applied.

The case-by-case approach is generally accepted, and seems to be the best approach for evaluating the considerable variety of genetic modifications in the various products. Moreover, by applying a case-by-case approach the latest scientific findings can be included in the evaluation, thereby guaranteeing maximum safety of the novel food products. One disadvantage of the case-by-case approach is that it may require more effort to safeguard uniformity of evaluation. Communication with the consumer could also be affected by this approach, and the evaluation procedure may take more time. It is feasible that once sufficient experience with the evaluation of novel food products has been gained, categories of products can be indicated which can be evaluated according to a simpler procedure if knowledge on product and insert is sufficient.

Classical animal feeding trials are not very adequate when complex novel foods are involved. Most advisory reports advocate a more analytical approach, but the limited knowledge of plant physiology and compositional variation may cause some major problems in that case. It can therefore be concluded that the introduction of novel foods derived from genetically modified organisms urges the toxicologist to develop new, simple concepts that can deal with transgenic complex foods. It is likely that such concepts should consist of both analytical and (new) toxicological methods, including *in vitro* systems. In addition, databases on the composition of food-graded species will have to be set up in order to perform risk analyses more efficiently. These databases will need to provide information on the presence and variation of macro- and micronutrients and natural toxins in food-graded species, including the different varieties.

In some experimental disciplines, additional fundamental research is necessary in order to improve risk evaluations procedures. Increased research efforts are especially necessary in the immunotoxicological, gut toxicological, and fundamental molecular biological (especially with respect to gene regulation) disciplines. Improved knowledge of plant physiology is also of importance for the safety evaluation of new varieties. Finally, additional knowledge of the phenomenon of post-translation modification would be extremely valuable.

References

1. Doc. SN 2091/94, 8 april 1994, amended proposal (Com (93) 631 – COD 426).

2. OECD (1993) *Safety Evaluation of Foods Derived by Modern Biotechnology: Concepts and Principles.* Paris.

3. Kok, E.J. *Evaluation of strategies for food safety assessment of genetically modified agricultural products.* RIKILT-DLO-report 93.08. Wageningen, the Netherlands.

Limitations of Whole Food Feeding Studies in Food Safety Assessment

Bruce Hammond,[1] Steve G. Rogers, Roy L. Fuchs

Monsanto Company
United States

Limitations of whole food feeding studies in food safety assessment

The utility of feeding complex mixtures to animals as in whole food feeding studies for safety assessment has been addressed by various scientific groups. This issue first arose during the safety assessment of irradiated foods. Initial efforts by FDA and industry to establish safety relied upon the use of traditional feeding studies in animals. Hundreds of animal feeding studies were conducted during the 1960s and 1970s with various irradiated foodstuffs. In 1981, FDA established the Irradiated Foods Task Group. This group of scientists reviewed these data and concluded that animal feeding studies have limited sensitivity to detect small changes in food. Based on these experiences, food scientists and nutritionists have recommended against the routine use of whole food feeding studies in safety assessment of foods derived from genetically modified plants. In the monograph published by the International Food Biotechnology Council (IFBC) on assessing the safety of foods produced by genetic modification, whole food feeding studies were not normally recommended. IFBC stated that whole food feeding studies, if undertaken, should be of relatively short duration to avoid the confounding factors such as nutritional imbalances which may develop after prolonged feeding. Similarly, the 1992 FDA Food Policy (published 29 May 1992) cautioned against the routine use of whole feeding studies for safety assessment of genetically modified food. We have conducted a number of short-term animal feeding studies to assess the wholesomeness of different foods/feeds derived from genetically modified and non-modified plants and have concluded that compositional analysis, comparing the levels of nutrients and toxicants, is of more value for assessing potential changes in food wholesomeness.

Introduction

Advances in biotechnology have made it possible to selectively introduce new traits into food crops that impart desirable agronomic properties. These properties include protection against insect pests and pathogens, alternative methods for weed control through tolerance to herbicides, delayed ripening of fruits and vegetables to enhance flavor and storage stability, and increased solids (e.g. starch) production in potatoes that reduces fat content of french fries and potato chips.[1] Other possibilities include increasing the nutrient value of foods, decreasing the levels of endogenous anti-nutrients and allergens. The introduction of new

---

[1] corresponding author

traits into food crops is accelerated over that which has been historically possible through conventional breeding techniques since it is possible to selectively introduce single specific traits into plants.

As these crops are beginning to enter the marketplace, the public wants reassurance that new varieties of food crops developed through genetic engineering are as safe and nutritious as those developed through conventional breeding. Although this assurance is seldom available for foods derived from conventional less selective breeding, regulatory agencies that have oversight of food safety have developed decision tree guidelines for assessing the safety and wholesomeness of these new varieties of food crops. The intent of this paper is to evaluate the usefulness of whole food feeding studies for the evaluation of wholesomeness and safety assessment of new crop varieties. Reference will be made to the positions taken by various regulatory and scientific groups on whole food feeding studies based in part on past experience gained through testing of irradiated foods. The approach used by Monsanto to assess the wholesomeness and safety of new varieties of food crops will also be presented.

The use of animal studies to assess the wholesomeness of whole foods has been addressed by various scientific organizations. A group of academic and industry experts in food safety was assembled a few years ago to provide a "comprehensive, scientifically-based foundation for the safety evaluation of foods and food ingredients derived from genetically modified plants and microorganisms."[2] Designated as the International Food Biotechnology Council (IFBC), this group of scientists offered the following advice on whole food feeding studies: "When genetic and compositional data, coupled with available toxicologic information, do not suffice to establish the safety of the food, IFBC recommends limited feeding studies in animals... Longer term toxicological studies on whole foods are typically insensitive and beset with confounding factors. They are rarely to be recommended, and when unavoidable, should be undertaken only with the most careful design and precautions".[2]

A report of a joint FAO/WHO (Food and Agricultural Organization/World Health Organization) consultation made a similar recommendation regarding whole food testing. "The need for toxicity testing will be determined in part by the nature of the modified food plant. Molecular, biological, and chemical analysis should always be conducted before the need for animal testing is assessed. When the assessment of genetic and compositional changes does not provide a satisfactory basis for the safety evaluation, it may be necessary to test the whole food in animal tests. The nature and extent of such testing must then be carefully assessed in relation to the need to provide additional assurance of safety."[3]

In the latest draft of the United States Food and Drug Administration (FDA) "Redbook II", FDA scientists addressed the subject of safety evaluation of new varieties of crops prepared via genetic engineering. In regard to whole food feeding studies, FDA stated "Animal feeding trials of foods derived from new plant varieties are not conducted routinely ... unless testing may be needed to ensure safety." They advised developers that considered conducting wholesomeness testing of food that " ... animal tests on whole foods, which are complex mixtures, present problems that are not associated with traditional animal toxicology tests designed to assess the safety of single chemicals. ... When tests are contemplated, careful attention should be paid to the test protocol, taking into account such issues as nutritional balance and sensitivity."[4]

Guidelines designed to assess the safety of "novel" foods developed by the United Kingdom Advisory Committee on Novel Foods and Processes (ACNFP) addressed some of the technical problems of whole food feeding studies which will be addressed later.[5] Recently, the decision-tree approach provided in the aforementioned document was revised to include new varieties of food crops developed through genetic engineering.[6] Citing the example of a genetically modified tomato, the decision tree highlighted the kind of information needed for safety assessment which included a toxicology assessment scheme. The scheme provided for the conduct of a 90 day toxicology study and genotoxicity tests if the genetic change introduced a "new chemical entity", and there was no existing toxicology data on the "entity". The "entity" was not defined. It is assumed that in the majority of cases, the "entity" would not include the protein expression product(s) of the cloned gene(s). In most cases, it would be exceedingly difficult and costly to obtain sufficient quantities of protein expression product to carry out a 90 day feeding study. Secondly, such testing in most cases would provide little useful information and would be a waste of animals. The digestive tract is designed to degrade ingested protein. Feeding the protein expression product to animals would most likely produce no detectable adverse effects. This has been the experience in the safety testing of enzymes used in food processing.[7] Secondly, there is no precedent that proteins such as enzymes, which are composed of common amino acids, would be genotoxic.[7] The proposed guideline revisions also states that the decision tree will be applied flexibly and the Committee is "willing to consider reasoned arguments as to why certain information may or not be relevant in individual cases."

Regulatory scientists in Canada cautioned that "The application of standard laboratory animal testing protocols to the toxicological evaluation of whole foods or major food constituents is fraught with technical difficulties."[8] While animal feeding studies would not normally be recommended, the Canadian draft guidelines left open the possibility that 90 day whole food feeding studies could be requested if the safety of the new variety of food was in question.

In the Netherlands, it has been recently proposed that all food crops with new traits introduced by genetic engineering be fed to rats for 90 days as a prerequisite for subsequent nutrition trials with humans.[9]

While the routine use of whole food toxicology studies is not generally recommended, some regulatory guidelines leave open the possibility that 90 day feeding studies could be required on a case-by-case basis. To understand why some have cautioned against the routine use of whole food feeding studies to assess safety/wholesomeness, the experiences gained from feeding irradiated foods to animals will be briefly reviewed.

Experience in testing irradiated foods

Beginning in the 1950s, there was considerable interest in using irradiation to control insect infestations in stored food, extend shelf life of fruits and vegetables, and reduce microbial contamination and spoilage of meat and other foods.[10] The FDA worked with the United States military, the U.S. Department of Agriculture (USDA) and interested parties in the private sector to assess the nutritional and toxicological aspects of irradiated food.[10] The FDA described their approach to assess the safety and wholesomeness of irradiated food as follows: "Initial efforts by FDA and industry to establish the safety of irradiated foods led to a scheme approximating traditional methods for evaluating substances added to the food supply. Because the radiation chemistry of foods was still largely unknown, and because irradiation produced many substances that were ill-defined, FDA required animal feeding studies to demonstrate that irradiated foods were safe. The initial philosophy of FDA scientists was to develop a core of wholesomeness studies on different types of foods to provide a matrix from which the safety of other foods could be deduced."[10] During the following 20-30 years, over 400 studies to assess the safety and wholesomeness of irradiated foods were completed.[10] Irradiated foods were subjected to traditional toxicology testing including subchronic and chronic feeding studies, reproduction and teratology testing etc. A few feeding studies with farm animals were also undertaken.

Many different kinds of irradiated food were tested over the years such as fruits (bananas, strawberries, mangoes); vegetables (onions, potatoes, peas, carrots, cabbage); grains (wheat flour); meat (fish, chicken, beef), beans (cocoa beans, coffee beans) and various combination of these and other foods. Such a large scale research effort was unprecedented as there had been little prior experience in feeding whole foods to laboratory animals.

FDA consulted with various committees of food safety experts over the ensuing years to review the data generated from whole food feeding tests and assess whether this information would resolve questions about the safety of irradiated foods. These groups concluded that there was no evidence that irradiation had produced adverse effects in animals fed irradiated foods.[10]

They also acknowledged technical problems in conducting these tests that sometimes limited their usefulness. In the early design of feeding studies, it was not appreciated that nutritional imbalances can result from feeding high levels of whole foods to animals. Using traditional toxicology testing methods, animals are usually fed exaggerated levels of test substances at levels at least 100 times higher than potential human exposure. When irradiated and non-irradiated whole foods were fed at exaggerated levels to animals for prolonged periods, adverse effects sometimes occurred which were due, in part, to nutritional imbalances (**Table 1**). These "secondary" adverse effects could mask potential toxicological manifestations produced by irradiation.[10] Furthermore, some foods which are wholesome for humans are not well tolerated when fed at exaggerated levels to animals.[11]

For whole food feeding studies, it was often not possible to feed animals 100 times the human equivalent dietary exposure. For example, "a rat that eats a diet containing 70 per cent wheat flour consumes only about 15 times the average human consumption in the United Kingdom (based on their relative body weights). In other studies, even by "concentrating" the intake of potatoes through partial drying, rats in feeding studies were consuming less than 25 times the average consumption in countries such as Germany or Ireland where this vegetable is a staple commodity in the national diet."[11]

Advances in analytical technology provided more sensitive and specific methods to assess the safety and wholesomeness of irradiated foods. The key safety issue involving irradiated foods was the possibility of generating radiolytic products in foods at levels that would be considered harmful. Prior to the advent of sensitive analytical tests, whole food feeding studies were the only tool available to monitor for potential adverse effects of irradiated foods. However, as discussed previously, whole food feeding tests have limited sensitivity to detect such changes due to the confounding effects from nutritional imbalances and inability to feed such foods at exaggerated levels. As the sensitivity and selectivity of analytical tests improved, it was possible to determine whether irradiation generated novel radiolytic products in food, or increased the level of endogenous radiolytic products such as those normally formed during cooking of food. Sensitive and specific analytical tests showed no evidence for the formation of measurable quantities (ppm levels) of radiolytic products of toxicological significance in food irradiated at doses below 1 kGy (100 krad). It was recognized that whole food feeding tests may not have the sensitivity to detect changes in radiolytic products at low ppm levels, even if hundreds of animals were used.[10] All of the analytical and animal feeding data was reviewed by a FDA consultant committee of scientific experts (Irradiated Foods Task Group) which concluded that "toxicological tests on foods irradiated at 1 kGy (100 krad) or below are not needed to support a conclusion that such foods are safe."[12]

In Europe, food scientists participating in the Joint FAO/IAEA/WHO Expert Committee on the Wholesomeness of Irradiated Food came to the same conclusions regarding animal feeding tests: "If irradiated foodstuffs are tested in animal studies, the level of potentially toxic radiation-induced compounds in the animal diet would probably not exceed 0.5 mg/kg. Effects due to such minute quantities would thus be undetectable in a standard animal experiment involving a maximum of 50 to 100 animals per group. For these reasons, little emphasis was placed by the Committee on continuing animal feeding studies as a basis for future acceptance of irradiated foods."[11]

It became apparent from review of all the data that whole food feeding studies were not sufficiently sensitive to detect whether small changes in the levels of radiolytic products were occurring in food. More reliance was placed on sensitive and specific analytical tests to detect any potential adverse changes in the food. While there was never any evidence that irradiation of food produced adverse effects in animals, secondary adverse effects sometimes occurred as a result of nutritional imbalances and/or biological or statistical variability.[13] Sometimes the cause of secondary adverse effects was not evident, requiring the study to be repeated. Sometimes hundreds or thousands of animals were used in repeat studies to determine if a previously reported adverse effect was reproducible or an artifact. This led to more costs and delays in reaching a decision about the safety of irradiated food. Militant critics of irradiated foods were never hesitant to reference any adverse results to advance their cause. The public became confused by the "apparent" conflicting data on food safety as reported by those who either opposed or supported the safety of irradiated foods.

Scientists who have reviewed the vast experiment in assessing the wholesomeness and safety of irradiated food were understandably hesitant to go down the same path for new varieties of food crops generated via genetic engineering. Leon Golberg, a respected expert in food safety once commented, "The solution attempted for the problem of irradiated foods has proved a colossal and costly failure. Feeding irradiated fruit salad to dogs has not established safety, nor has the vast exercise provided an advance in fundamental knowledge to serve as a springboard for further work."[14] Dr Golberg believed that it was essential to first identify, through analytical techniques, the chemical identity of food constituents of interest. Once this was done, one could better determine what, if any biological testing was needed to more fully understand the biologic activity of the constituent and its significance to food safety.

At Monsanto, we have taken a similar position in our assessment of the wholesomeness/safety of new varieties of food crops developed through genetic engineering. We rely primarily on the use of sensitive and specific analytical tests to detect any potential untoward changes that might have occurred in the food as a result of the genetic modification. The safety questions are different from irradiated foods which were concerned with the possible presence of harmful radiolytic products in food. The fundamental safety questions for food crops modified through genetic engineering are: 1) the safety of protein expression products of the introduced genes, and 2) the potential for unintended untoward (pleitrophic) effects resulting from insertion of the introduced gene(s).

Monsanto's approach to addressing these safety concerns is as follows:

1) Safety of the expressed protein(s) of introduced genes

a) The biological activity of the expressed protein must be defined and shown not to pose an unacceptable health risk if ingested.

Monsanto has introduced genes into plants that express proteins imparting the following functions:

i) Enzymes that catalyze metabolic reactions in plants such as degradation of ethylene which delays ripening of tomatoes, enhancement of starch synthesis in potatoes to decrease fat content in fried potatoes, tolerance to glyphosate (active ingredient of ROUNDUP®) herbicide providing alternative weed control options for farmers, etc.

ii) Proteins from the *Bacillus thuringiensis* (*Bt*) family of microorganisms that impart protection against specific plant pests. This family of proteins exhibit selective toxicity to certain insect pests that contain specific receptors on insect gut cells that permit the *Bt* protein to bind to and kill gut cells. This family of proteins are inactive in non-target insects, invertebrates and mammals since they lack the receptors on their gut cells.[15]

(iii) Marker proteins that facilitate the plant transformation process (a low frequency event) by selecting cells containing the introduced genes in culture. These markers can be proteins that impart tolerance to glyphosate, discussed above, or to antibiotics such as kanamycin.

The biologic activity of the expressed protein should be well understood. In the case of enzymes, the substrate and catalytic products should be defined. Where appropriate, the concentration of both the introduced protein and the metabolite products produced by the introduced protein (if an enzyme) in edible plant tissue should be measured. For example, the enzyme that imparts tolerance to glyphosate is involved in aromatic amino acid synthesis. This pathway is only present in plant tissue which contributes to the lack of toxicity of glyphosate to mammals and other non-plant life forms. No changes in the levels of individual or total aromatic acids were found in plant tissue expressing this enzyme.[16]

b) The source and genetic sequence of the cloned gene should be identified.

The source of the gene which is introduced into plants should be identified and the nucleic acid sequence of the gene determined.

Table 1
Examples of Adverse Effects from Feeding Animals Whole Foods

Food	Effect	Ref.
Onions	Rats and dogs fed up to 35% (dry weight) onions develop anemia from hemolysis of red blood cells. Rats fed for 90 days exhibit pigmentation of spleen, liver, kidney (hemosiderin?)	23
Potatoes	Rats fed boiled potatoes for 17 days developed enlarged caecums. Megacolon has been observed in rats fed high levels of modified starch.	24, 25
Wheat flour	Reduced breeding performance in multigeneration rat study fed 35% flour in diet. Survival of rats reduced significantly in chronic study.	26
Tomatoes	Mucosal necrosis/erosion of stomach in rats fed 30 gm/kg/day tomato paste by gavage for four weeks.	27
Beans	Rats fed beans (*Phaeseolus vulgaris*) only for 12 weeks developed emphysematous enlargements of air sacs in the lung.	28
Chili	Gavaging rats with 10% chili pepper solution for four weeks produced damage to the duodenal mucosa.	29
Macadamia nuts	Produce fever, partial paralysis, lameness in dogs lasting 12-24 hrs after ingestion.	30

c) **The amino acid sequence of the expressed protein should be confirmed to be the same as that predicted by the gene sequence.**

d) **The levels of expression of the cloned protein in edible plant tissue should be determined.**

   It has been our experience that the proteins are expressed at low levels in edible plant tissue. If the plant tissue (food) is heat processed and solvent extracted (as in the case of soybeans), the biologic activity of the expressed proteins is destroyed during the process.[16] Oils derived from soybeans and other seeds are essentially devoid of protein.[16]

e) **The amino acid sequence of the cloned protein should not be closely related to known allergens or toxins.**

   The amino acid sequence of the cloned protein is compared to sequences in computer protein data banks to confirm that it is not similar to known protein toxins or allergens. If the enzymatic function of the cloned protein is the same as enzymes endogenously present in food, the sequence homology of the proteins is compared to establish a basis of historical consumption.

f) **The expressed proteins should be readily degraded by proteases in the gastrointestinal tract.**

   Since the proteins encoded by the genes introduced into plants are expressed at low levels in plant tissue, the gene used for the plant transformation is typically introduced into a microbial system where the protein is expressed at a high level, purified, and shown to be functionally and structurally equivalent to the protein expressed in the genetically engineered plant. The protein is incubated in simulated digestive fluids to assess its potential digestibility if ingested. To date, eight different proteins that have been expressed in plants have been tested in the simulated digestion study. All, as expected, are readily digested in this test system.[16]

g) **The protein products of cloned genes must not be toxic when administered orally at exaggerated dosages to mice.**

   The acute toxicity of the protein is tested in mice. Proteins that are toxic manifest adverse effects following acute exposure.[7,17,18] Toxic proteins produced by bacterial pathogens are generally toxic at µg/kg oral dosages. For example, *Staphylococcal aureus* enterotoxins A&B produce emesis and diarrhea in primates following acute oral doses of 0.9 µg/kg in primates and ~ 1.5 µg/kg in man.[19] *Clostridium perfringens* toxin produces diarrhea in mice at an acute oral dosage of 100 µg/kg; and gastrointestinal upset in man at ~ 150 µg/kg.[20] A common feature of some bacterial protein toxins is their heat stability and resistance to proteases such as trypsin. The stability of these bacterial protein toxins contributes to their toxicity as they would survive longer in the gut. In contrast, the protein expression products of genes introduced into plants by Monsanto are not stable as they are both heat labile and readily degraded by proteases, like most food proteins. They exhibit no toxicity when administered orally to mice at acute dosages of 100,000 to 1,000,000 µg/kg. These dosages are much higher than those which produce adverse effects for microbial protein toxins and represent 1000 to 100,000 fold or greater safety factors for estimated human consumption. The lack of toxicity observed in acute gavage studies in mice administered the aforementioned protein expression products was based on in-life observations, body weight and food consumption measurements and a thorough necropsy seven days post-dosing. If any unusual findings are observed in tissues at necropsy, these are saved for microscopic examination. The proteins are expressed at ppm levels in raw food. They are largely destroyed in processed food and would pose no meaningful health risk even if ingested.

We believe the aforementioned testing scheme for the protein expression product(s) of cloned genes provides ample assurance that the proteins pose no meaningful risks to human health.

2) Use of sensitive and specific analytical tests to address unintended (pleitrophic) effects

Plants that are consumed for food provide varying amounts of the daily requirement for important nutrients. In an accompanying Monsanto paper in this session, a list of important nutrients present in soybeans is provided.[16] Glyphosate-tolerant soybeans were analyzed for all of these nutrients and the results compared to those obtained for the parental, non-transformed line from which the modified variety was derived. Both the parental and transformed variety were grown at the same time and in the same field test plots to minimize potential variability in nutrients resulting from differing agronomic conditions. The analytical results were also compared to published data to be certain the nutrient levels were within expected ranges. The same process was followed for important endogenous anti-nutrient components present in soybeans (e.g. trypsin inhibitors, lectins, phytoestrogens, phytates).[21] Natural anti-nutrient components provide protection against plant pathogens.[22] As before, the levels of anti-nutrient components in the modified plant are compared to its parental control and the published literature to make sure there have been no meaningful changes in endogenous toxicants. Processing fractions of the food crop may also be analyzed to verify that the parameters measured are within accepted limits, e.g. amino acid content of protein soy isolate, lipid fractionation of processed soybean oil, etc.[16]

3) **Selective use of wholesomeness tests**

These studies are conducted as needed and are supportive of more sensitive and specific analytical testing discussed previously. The wholesomeness of the food modified to contain new traits is compared to that of the parental non-modified line grown at the same time and in the same field plots. Generally, these feeding trials are conducted with farm animals simulating commercial feeding practices. For example, 98 per cent of soybeans are fed to farm animals. Thus, our glyphosate-tolerant soybeans have been fed to chickens, catfish and dairy cows. The soybeans were formulated into the diets at commercial application rates. The chicken and catfish studies are the most sensitive tests to detect changes in nutritional value, since these animals experience approximately 700 per cent growth during the feeding trials (e.g. a 40 gram broiler chicken at study start weighs ~ 2000 grams at study termination). Animal feeding trials are not carried out on crops that are modified to contain new traits via traditional plant breeding practices. However, it is recognized that the introduction of new traits into food crops by genetic engineering or biotechnology is sometimes considered to be more controversial than the use of traditional plant breeding techniques. The conduct of appropriate animal feeding trials provides an added safety assurance at this time. If experience shows that such testing is not needed to confirm safety, these tests should be eliminated.

For modified food crops that are consumed by humans, we have fed the crop to rats at up to 25 times the highest estimated human exposure (if feasible). The trials are conducted over four weeks with ten rats/sex/group. The amount of food administered is not excessive, to avoid nutritional imbalances discussed previously. For whole foods (potatoes, tomatoes) we introduce an entire vegetable in the cage with the addition of the laboratory chow. This allows the rat to receive its typical diet plus the vegetable. It has been our experience that rats eat usual amounts of rodent chow and a whole tomato or potato every two to three days. In the case of seed meal, which is better incorporated in the diet (e.g. processed soybean meal, corn meal), we have substituted modified meal for non-modified meal in the rodent diet at commercial rates of incorporation. The modified and non-modified (parental line) meal is analyzed for proximate composition (protein, fat, ash, moisture, etc.) and the rodent diets are formulated to be isonitrogenous. Since the animal tests insensitive to small changes in the food, the wholesomeness parameters examined include daily observations for health, weekly body weight and food consumption, and a thorough gross necropsy at the end of the four-week test. If any unusual findings are observed at necropsy, tissues are saved for microscopic examination. These rat feeding studies are not designed to be toxicology tests, but are intended to compare the wholesomeness of modified to non-modified (parental line) food. These studies provide supplementary information to the extensive analytical testing discussed above.

Conclusion

The safety assessment strategy that has been presented provides a rational means to assess the wholesomeness and safety of new varieties of food crops developed by genetic engineering. Primary reliance is given to sensitive and specific analytical tests to assess for unintended effects and to characterize the gene insert. Additional information on the biologic function and safety of the protein expression product is also provided. Whole food feeding studies would not be sensitive enough to pick up the potential occurrence of small unintended effects; these could be better detected analytically. Animal tests would also not detect potential adverse effects from protein expression products, since they are present in low (ppm) amounts in raw food and are largely destroyed in processed food. However, where appropriate, whole food feeding studies can provide supporting evidence of food wholesomeness and confirmation that no significant unintended effects occurred in the food crop.

References

1. Gasser, C.S. and Fraley, R.T. (1989) Genetically engineering plants for crop improvement. *Science* 244:1293-1299.

2. International Food Biotechnology Council (1990). Biotechnologies and food: assuring the safety of foods produced by genetic modification. *Regulatory Toxicology and Pharmacology* 12:S1-S196).

3. *Strategies for assessing the safety of foods produced by biotechnology* (1991). Report of a Joint FAO/WHO Consultation. World Health Organization.

4. Toxicological Principles for the Safety Assessment of Direct Food Additives and Color Additives Used in Food (1993). "Redbook II" Draft. US Food and Drug Administration, Center for Food Safety and Applied Nutrition.

5. Guideline on the Assessment of Novel Foods and Processes (ACNFP) (1991). Department of Health. Report on Health and Social Subjects No. 38. HMSO, London. ISBN 0 11 321336 0.

6. A Structured Approach for the Safety Assessment of Novel Foods and Processes: Revision to Chapter 4 of the ACNFP's Guideline. 7 July 1994.

7. Pariza, M.W. and Foster, E.M. (1983) Determining the Safety of Enzymes Used in Food Processing. *J Food Protection* 46:453-468.

8. Draft Guidelines for the Safety Assessment of Novel Foods. Food Directorate, Health Protection Branch, Health Canada. October 1993.

9. Health Council of the Netherlands HCN (1992) Safety of food produced by new biotechnology. Publication No. 92/O3E, The Hague.

10. Pauli, G.H. and Takeguchi, C.A. (1986) Irradiation of Foods – An FDA Perspective. Foods Reviews International 2(1):79-107.

11. Elias, P. (1980) The Wholesomeness of Irradiated Food. *Ecotoxicology and Environmental Safety* 4:172-183.

12. Irradiation in the Production, Processing, and Handling of Food. *Federal Register* Vol. 51, No. 75, 18 April 1986.

13. Radiological and Toxicological Safety of Irradiated Foods. In: *Safety of Irradiated Foods* (J.F. Diehl, ed.). Marcel Dekker, New York (1990).

14. Golberg, L. (1970) Chemical and Biochemical Implications of Human and Animal Exposure to Toxic Substances in Food. *Pure and Applied Chemistry* 21:309-330.

15. Laird, M., Lacey, L.A. and Davidson, E.W. (eds.) (1989) *Safety of Microbial Insecticides*. CRC Press, Inc., Baco Raton, Florida.

16. Fuchs, R.L., et al. Safety Evaluation of Glyphosate-tolerant Soybeans (this Workshop).

17. Sjoblad, R.D., McClintock, J.T. and Engler, R. (1992) Toxicological Considerations for Protein Components of Biological Pesticide Products. *Regulatory Toxicology and Pharmacology* 15:3-9.

18. Jones, D.D and Maryanski, J.H. (1991) Safety Considerations in the Evaluation of Transgenic Plants for Human Foods. In: *Risk Assessment in Genetic Engineering* (M.A. Levin and H.S. Strauss, eds.). McGraw-Hill, New York.

19. Schantz, E.J., et al. (1965) Purification of Staphylococcal Enterotoxin B". *Biochemistry* 4:1011-1016.

20. Labbe, R. (1989) Clostridium perfringens". In: *Foodborne Bacterial Pathogens* (M.P. Doyle, ed.). Marcell Dekker, New York.

21. Leiner, I.E. (1994) Implications of Antinutritional Components in Soybean Foods". Critical reviews in *Food Science and Nutrition* 34(1):31-67.

22. Ames, B.N. (1983) Dietary Carcinogens and Anticarcinogens. Oxygen radicals and degenerative diseases. *Science* 221:1256-1264.

23. *Wholesomeness of Irradiated Food with Special Reference to Wheat, Potatoes and Onions*. Report of a Joint FAO/IAEA/WHO Expert Committee. World Health Organization Technical Report Series No. 451 (1970).

24. Mathers, J.C. and Dawson, L.D. (1991) Large bowel fermentation in rats eating processed potatoes. *British Journal of Nutrition* 466:313-329).

25. Roe, J.C. (1989) What is wrong with the way we test chemicals for carcinogenic activity. In: *Advances in Applied Toxicology*. (A.D. Dayan and A.J. Paine, eds.). Taylor and Francis Ltd., London.

26. Tinsley, I.J., Bone, J.F. and Bubl, E.C. (1965) The Growth, Reproduction, Longevity, and Histopathology of Rats Fed Gamma-Irradiated Flour. *Toxicology and Applied Pharmacology* 7:71-78.

27. *Food Chemical News*, 6 Sept. 1993, p. 18.

28. Palacek, F. (1969) Pulmonary Damage in Rats Fed by Beans (*Phaseolus vulgaris*). *Experientia* 25:285.

29. Jang, J.J., et. al. (1992) A 4-Week Feeding Study of Ground Red Chili (*Capsicum anuum*) in Male B6C3F1 Mice. *Food Chemistry and Toxicology* 30:783-787.

30. Personnel communication from William B. Buck, DVM., University of Illinois National Animal Poison Control Center, Urbana, Illinois (1994).

The Concept of Substantial Equivalence: Toxicological Testing of Novel Foods

Norman R. Lazarus

Department of Health
United Kingdom

Introduction

The concept of *substantial equivalence* has been well enunciated by the OECD.[1] The idea behind the concept was to develop an approach in evaluating novel foods that was not encumbered by a prescribed set of testing. This approach is different from that used for Food Additives and Contaminants.[2] However neither *substantial* nor *equivalence* have dimensions. Thus a food which is 99 per cent the same as a readily available product, i.e. substantially equivalent but contains a new toxic principle, may require extensive testing. Whereas a new food with only 70 per cent correspondence may require little testing especially if the difference is in nutritional components can readily be replaced by a mixed diet. Thus it may be expected that the concept will not be very useful in predicting which products will require substantial testing. In this paper some examples of the application of the OECD concept to evaluation of some novel foods will be presented. The list is not intended to be exhaustive. Some of the foods under discussion have been evaluated by the UK Advisory Committee for Novel Foods and Processes (ACNFP). Others have been evaluated by similar bodies in other countries.

Lupins

The seeds of the narrow leaved lupin (*Lupinus angustifolius*) and the white lupin (*Lupinus albus*) have been used in human diets although not in the UK. The seeds of most varieties contain high levels of alkaloids but recently narrow leaved lupins have been bred which have low alkaloid levels in their seeds. For these plants Phomopsins are likely fungal contaminants. These mycotoxins are responsible for a disease in animals called lupinosis. They are hepatotoxins.[6]

Toxicological considerations involve questions on the nutritional composition of the seeds, alkaloid concentrations and contaminating mycotoxins. The nutritional component can be evaluated by feeding semi-synthetic diets to animals in which general nutritional state and growth will be important end points. Other tests will involve mutagenicity of the alkaloids and their effects in a multigeneration study. *In vivo* tests in 15 day old rats can be used to detect Phomopsins (see **Table 2**).

Table 1
Foods Under Discussion

Product type	Example
Seeds	Lupins
Fat replacer	Sucrose polyester
Synthetic oils	Triglyceride
GMO enzyme	Chymosin
Probiotics	Lactobacillus GG

If the concept of *substantial equivalence* is applied it is not sure whether lupins are substantially different from other products on the market. While lupin proteins may have different physico-chemical characteristics to other proteins it is probable that their amino acid composition is similar. Thus if the composition of the protiens are known there should be little necessity for extensive nutritional studies. Tests on alkaloid and mycotoxin contamination would normally be required whether the concept was applied or not. Substantial equivalence does not appear to be helpful in formulating what testing is required.

Fat replacer

Recently the idea of replacing fats in the diet with non-absorbable non-metabolisable substances has been in vogue. The molecule that is currently under scrutiny by a number of regulatory authorities is a polysucrose.

Toxicological considerations revolve around the effects of such a molecule on GIT absorption and/secretion, possible GIT pathology and whether the molecule is absorbed in small but toxicologically significant quantities.

The use of animals in an initial assessment of the polysucrose on the absorption of fat soluble molecules is mandatory before safety clearance can be given. If the molecule is not absorbed then further more extensive toxicity studies may not be required.

This substance has no *equivalent* in current dietary intakes and would require animal toxicity testing before undergoing trials in humans. Once again it does nor require the annunciation of a concept to decide whether testing is required or not **(Table 3)**.

GMO chymosin

This enzyme is identical to naturally occurring enzyme. If a pure enzyme is available then the concept of *substantial equivalence* can be invoked with no further testing. The presence of contaminating molecules may require animal testing[4] **(Table 4)**.

Table 2
Lupins for Lupin Flour (*L. augustifolus*, *L. albus*)

Toxicological considerations

1. Nutritional composition of the seeds

2. Alkaloids in flour

    lupanine   13 hydroxylupanine   augustifoline   isolupanine

3. Contaminating mycotoxins

Use of animals	End-point
1. Semi-synthetic diets using lupin flour as a protein source (55.5g lupin/100g test diet)	growth general nutrition
2. Spiking of synthetic diets with different concentrations of purified alkaloids	repeat dose study mutagenicity multigeneration

Conclusions

In general, the introduction of novel proteins that make up a substantial portion of the diet would tend to generate much discussion on the wholesomeness of the proteins. However, unless these proteins contain amino acids not present in other proteins, these studies are not very worthwhile.

Substantial equivalence, for reasons stated in the text, is not a very helpful concept to apply.

Table 3
Sucrose Polyester – Non-absorbable Fat Replacer

Toxicological considerations

1. May interfere with GIT absorption and/or secretion

2. GIT pathology

3. Truly non-absorbable?

Use of animals	**End-point**
1. Absorption studies	blood, urine, lymphoid tissue
2. Assessment of effects on fat soluble components of the diet	vitamins, billary excretion
3. Pathology in GIT	histology

Conclusions

Testing in animals can give many pointers to the potential toxic effects of these types of compounds and confirm lack of absorption.

Human studies are paramount because of the differing vitamin status of selected populations.

Concept of substantial equivalence does not apply since products are unique.

Table 4
Synthetic Triglyceride

Toxicological considerations

1. Is toxicity associated with the increased intake of saturated fatty acid which may already be in the diet?

Use of animals	End-point
1. Feeding studies	metabolism, digestion growth, organ toxicity

Conclusions

Animals may be used in a preliminary screen for effects. Human studies are paramount because of possible effects of long chain fatty acids on clotting, etc. in susceptible populations. The application of substantial equivalence would at first glance suggest little testing is required. However, the concerns about "nutritional toxicology" would suggest extensive clinical testing. The concept is not useful here.

Lactobacillus GG

The lactobacilli are a family of bacteria which produce lactic acid as a byproduct of their growth. Lactobacillus strains are present naturally at low concentrations in certain constituents of the UK diet. Lactobacillus GG was specifically isolated as a starter culture for fermented products such as yoghurt. Safety evaluation of this product concluded that there were no reasons why foods containing Lactobacillus GG should not be consumed providing an agreed specification was met.[5] There has been a tendency to make therapeutic claims about these Lactobacilli. Therapeutic claims for food are not allowed in the UK.

The concept of *substantial equivalence* may be useful in the safety evaluation of this food (see **Table 5**).

Novel synthetic food components

Since novel chemical processes can give rise to foods that have novel structures[3] it may be useful, in this final example, to do a thought experiment. Let us suppose that a novel synthetic oil is synthesized. The only difference between this oil and others already on the market is that it contains a slightly higher concentration of a saturated fatty acid.

On superficial examination it may appear that this food is substantially equivalent to others already on the market. However it is well documented that an increased intake in saturated fats can increase the thrombotic potential especially in an at risk population. Animal studies probably will not be useful models in answering these types of nutritional toxicological questions. Animals can be used to answer the broad question of whether increased consumption of a normal dietary component can have untoward side effects. However the use of animals may be limited since the effects of long chain saturated fatty acids may have unique effects in the human population.

The fact that the components of the triglyceride are *substantially equivalence* to what is already in the diet should have allowed for limited animal and/or human studies. This will certainly not be the case.

Conclusions

It is apparent even from this short list of novel foods that certain general conclusions can be made:

a) Because *substantial equivalence* has no dimensions it cannot be predicted which novel foods will require substantial toxicological testing in animals

b) Depending upon the nature of the novel food, the usefulness of the concept ranges from useful to negligible.

c) The number and range of tests will be determined by the nature of the product under consideration.

d) A checklist of animal toxicological procedures is inappropriate for novel foods.

Table 5
Probiotics lactobacillus GG
Live Strain of a Lactobacillus (Yoghurts, etc.)

Toxicological considerations

1. GIT colonization

Use of animals

1. Nil

Human studies directed to colonization in human gut.

Concept of substantial equivalence may be useful.

Table 6
GMO Enzyme Chymosin

Toxicological considerations

1. Nil on pure enzyme

Use of animals   **End-point**

1. Nil   —

Conclusions

Provided the enzyme is in a reasonably pure state, this product may be said to be substantially equivalent to what is already available.

Application of substantial equivalence is trivial.

References

1. OECD (1993) *Safety Evaluation of Foods Derived by Modern Biotechnology: Concepts and Principles*. Paris.

2. WHO (1970) *Principles for the Safety Assessment of Food Additives and Contaminants; Environmental Health Criteria* 70.

3. *Journal of the American College of Toxicology* (1991) 10(3):323-367.

4. ACNFP Annual Report 1989. MAFF Publications, London SE99 7TP.

5. ACNFP Annual Report 1993. MAFF Publications, London SE99 7TP.

6. Keeler and Tu, eds. (1991) *Phomopsins: Antimicotubule Mycotoxins in Toxicology of Plant and Fungal Compounds*. Marcel Dekker, 371-395.

Dietary Assessment Related to the Safety Evaluation of Foods

Michael Nelson

Department of Nutrition and Dietetics
King's College London

The safety evaluation of foods, including evaluation of microbiological and chemical contamination and the potential hazards related to novel foods, must at some point embrace an assessment of the amounts likely to be consumed by individuals within the population. The assessment of intake, or "exposure", is fraught with difficulties, and I would like to talk first of all about the context in which dietary assessment takes place in relation to food safety evaluation, second about the errors likely to be associated with dietary assessment and how to cope with them, and third about novel methods of assessment which are intended to improve the quality of dietary data collected from individuals.

The context of dietary assessment

In order to choose an appropriate method for dietary assessment, the context in which the assessment is to take place must be considered. In this instance, we are concerned about the risks associated with the ingestion of potentially toxic substances, or the evaluation of the effects of consumption of novel foods. The assumption at the outset is either that the substance is known to be harmful (a particular microorganism or toxin, or a chemical contaminant introduced at production, processing, or during storage), or that the consumption of a novel substance is potentially harmful and its consumption requires monitoring for ill effects.

There must be a clearly defined relationship between the exposure and the outcome. In reality, the measurements that are made are only approximations of the real values. It is incumbent upon those who make these measurements to satisfy themselves as to the validity of the measures. An attenuated assessment may lead to a false estimate of a safe threshold or maximum allowable residue level. Assessment in relation to chronic outcomes which may take years to develop requires appropriate follow-up and monitoring of populations whose exposure may change with time. Within the population, there may be vulnerable groups (children, pregnant women, the elderly) or at-risk groups (diabetics and consumption of artificial sweeteners, patients with a history of hepatitis in relation to exposure to aflatoxin and risk of liver cancer) whose diets need close monitoring. There may also be enthusiastic consumers (e.g. health food shoppers, winkle pickers) whose dietary habits may lead to ingestion of foods whose average consumption in the population is minimal. Close monitoring of the levels of harmful substances in foods rather than identification of the consumers *per se* may be the most appropriate approach to food safety for particular foodstuffs eaten by a small but enthusiastic minority. And there may be critical periods of exposure (e.g. retinol in the first trimester of pregnancy, leading to increased teratogenesis) which need to be identified. An accurate knowledge of the levels of intake and likely associated outcomes is required in order to be able to undertake quantitative risk assessment or to calculate population attributable risks.

Validity, reliability, and errors of measurement

Validity (the extent to which a measurement measures what it purports to measure) and reliability (or reproducibility, or repeatability – the extent to which a measurement produces the same result in the same situation) provide measures of the usefulness of data. Reliability does not imply validity. We need to establish the relationship between what we measure and the relevant true values, be they of exposure or outcome. This can be achieved in part by a detailed assessment of the errors associated with the measurement. Proportional and constant biases will distort our impression of the cutoff points for threshold, or will inflate or deflate true dose-response relationships. If known, they can be corrected for in the same way for every measurement. Random error is often associated with biological or day to day variation within subjects, and can be accounted for by taking sufficient number of measurements in order to allow the errors to cancel each other out. Measurements which differ in their bias from one subject to another will lead to differential misclassification: some subjects will be seen to have an exposure or outcome different to other subjects when in reality the exposure or outcome is the same in both groups. This type of bias is likely to lead to an incorrect interpretation of exposure-outcome relationships. In some circumstances, if the extent of the bias is known, or the characteristics of those subjects who are most likely to provide biased data are recognized, it may allow for an analysis of the data which is corrected for these errors.

Tools for validation

In recent years, three techniques have been used to assess the validity of measures of diet which were previously thought to be accurate. These techniques are doubly-labelled water, nitrogen excretion in validated 24-hour urine collections, and estimated energy intake/requirement ratios. By excluding subjects who under-report their intakes, the true levels associated with measured outcomes are more likely to be identified.

Doubly-labelled water (with deuterium and oxygen-18) can be used to provide an indirect but very accurate assessment of energy expenditure. This can be compared with estimates of energy intake based on diet records or recall. Disagreements between the two measures allow the identification of those likely to under-report their true consumption. This typically includes subjects who are overweight. Their exposures are therefore likely to be underestimated if based on unvalidated dietary assessments. With this method of validation, subjects may distort their reported consumption of foods which are not important sources of energy without being detected. The technique is very expensive and expertise in the analysis of the material is extremely limited.

More feasible is assessment of urinary nitrogen. Subjects in nitrogen balance typically excrete about 81 per cent of dietary nitrogen in the urine. Subjects whose estimated dietary nitrogen is less than their urinary nitrogen are likely to be under-reporting. The completeness of the 24-hour urine collection can be assessed by administering PABA (para-amino-benzoic acid) in split doses three times a day. PABA is rapidly absorbed in the gut and excreted unaltered in the urine. Subjects whose urine contains at least 85 per cent of the administered dose can be regarded as having provided a complete sample.

Where biochemical techniques are not available, identification of subjects with the most severe under-reporting can be obtained by comparing estimates of energy intake with estimates of requirement based on age, gender and body weight. An intake less than 1.2

times the estimated basal metabolic rate (BMR) is not sufficient to maintain a free-living person in energy balance. This technique does not identify subjects with higher energy requirements whose intake/BMR ratio may be greater than 1.2.

Dietary assessment techniques in post-marketing monitoring and surveillance

While average population exposures can be assessed using data obtained at the national level, this is rarely sufficiently accurate to be used for food safety monitoring. Data at the household or individual level are required.

Household acquisition data has the strengths of national representation (which makes it appropriate as a basis for total diet studies to assess average levels of contaminants) and will provide useful information about patterns of consumption regionally, or between household types, or over time. The main weaknesses have to do with the assessment of foods which are eaten away from home, or foods (such as sweets, soft drinks and alcoholic beverages) which usually fall outside the purview of the respondent. There is general evidence of an over-reporting bias, which may be greater in low income than high income households. This may obscure some differences (in insecticides associated with fruit consumption, for example) and over-emphasize others (e.g. sugar intake). Apart from total diet studies, or studies with concomitant analysis of specific contaminants, all forms of dietary recording or recall rely on food composition data for their interpretation in relation to food safety.

Assessment of individual intakes, whether prospectively or retrospectively, also relies on food composition data, with the exception of duplicate diet studies. Every method has its particular strengths, but they all share many weaknesses. The intensity of the work involved for subjects completing records of consumption, and the memory and conceptualization skills needed by those asked to recall their consumption, lead inevitably to differential misclassification according to ability. There are also likely to be distortions of diet related to the recording or recall processes themselves.

Recent developments in dietary assessment methods

There have been several recent attempts to overcome some of the problems inherent in dietary assessment. The thrust has been to reduce respondent burden, provide better tools for assessment, or develop techniques which improve reporting (and to understand the errors associated with their use).

PETRA

PETRA is a system based on battery-operated electronic scales with a built in tape recorder. Subjects place a plate or container on the pan of the scales, press a button on the front of the device, and describe verbally what is present, e.g. "empty plate". They then place food on the plate, press the button, and describe the food. The tape thus keeps a record of the weight recorded at each press of the button, and a related verbal description. The tape is then transcribed using a master console, and the weights and descriptions written out and then analysed using conventional dietary computer software.

The device does not allow subjects to see the weights of what they are eating – there is no visual display of weights. There is no need to keep a manual record of consumption or transcribe weights from a scale display to a record book. It therefore helps to overcome some important problems relating to the skills of the subjects. It does require extensive transcription and decoding once the tape has been recorded. In comparison with battery operated digital scales for use with a record book, it is expensive.

IDA

IDA (Integrated Dietary Analysis) combines:

- a hand-held computer which integrates with weighing scales, if available, to provide a computer readable record of food consumption. It therefore avoids the necessity for writing records, and saves enormously on transcription time as the diet data does not have to be entered by the researcher;

- computer software for complex analyses according to time and place of eating, time of day, type of subject, etc.; and

- output in the form of an SPSS programme, which allows rapid integration of dietary data with other data collected.

The system is designed specifically for use in research, but also has applications in clinical settings. It is ideally suited to rapid recording and assessment of dietary data without the need for data transcription.

Food photography

Dietary recall requires subjects to conceptualize their diet in terms of frequency and amounts of foods consumed. The ability to conceptualize portion size and describe amounts clearly varies between subjects. A standard set of food photographs has been developed to assist with the description of foods which are difficult to describe in household measures. Research on the value of photographs in improving estimates of nutrient intake show clearly the size of the benefit associated with the use of photographs, and also the types of error associated with their use. Briefly, a series of eight photographs of portion size ranging from the 5th to the 95th centile consumed by British adults increases by 10 per cent the number of subjects correctly classified in thirds of the distribution of nutrient intakes compared with "standard" portion sizes or verbal descriptions in household measures. Single photographs of average portions (where subjects were asked to state their consumption in terms of the fraction or multiple of the amount depicted in the photograph) were less useful than a series of eight photographs. Small portion sizes tend to be overestimated and large portion sizes underestimated. Women and older people tended to overestimate portion size, and men and overweight subjects tended to underestimate their portion sizes. An atlas of sets of eight photographs of 76 foods is currently in preparation and should be available from early 1995.

Future work on dietary assessment in relation to food safety

There is a need to harmonize methods across European countries. Some effort in this direction has already begun, e.g. EPIC, EUROFOODS. New methods of dietary assessment and evaluation are being developed (e.g. IDA, PETRA, food photographs), but more are required that reduce respondent burden and consequent misclassification. New statistical techniques are being developed for combining results from several assessments to improve classification of subjects. In many circumstances the deficiencies of one method for one population subgroup may be made up for using an alternative method. Lastly, a more widespread and improved understanding of differential misclassification, how it arises, and how it affects interpretation of food safety issues is needed.

FOOD SAFETY EVALUATION

The context of dietary assessment:

1. Is there a substance known to be harmful?

    - Microbiological: organism or toxin
    - Chemical contaminant: production, processing, storage
    - Novel food

2. What is the relationship between exposure and outcome?

    - Threshold effect
    - Dose-response
    - Outcome measure: acute, chronic

3. What is the level of exposure?

    - Population average
    - Vulnerable groups
    - At-risk groups
    - Enthusiastic consumers
    - Window of effect

4. What is the risk associated with exposure in human populations?

DIETARY ASSESSMENT TECHNIQUES

Point of measurement:

    I   Domestic

    II National

Post-marketing monitoring and surveillance:

    III Household acquisition

    IV Household inventory

    V   Individual

HOUSEHOLD ACQUISITION/INVENTORY

Strengths:

- Nationally representative (total diet study)
- Variations by region, income, age, etc.
- Time trends

Limitations:

- Response rate
- Acquisition versus inventory
- Home food versus food away
- Soft drinks, sweets, alcoholic beverages
- Bias, especially by income
- No individuals
- Food composition tables

DIETARY ASSESSMENT OF INDIVIDUALS

Prospective (record) ("current")

    Duplicate diet
    Weighed inventory
    Household measures
    Food checklist

Retrospective (recall) ("usual" or "past")

    Diet history
    24 hour recall
    Questionnaire
    (Frequency/amount)

Strengths:

    Current, observable, direct, individual

    Quick, cheap, low cost and motivation

Limitations:

    Skills and motivation needed
    Labour intensive
    Distortion
    Differential misclassification
    Food composition tables

    Memory, conceptual, and interviewer bias
    Regular habits
    No daily variation
    Food composition tables

VALIDITY

The extent to which a measurement measures what it purports to measure

RELIABILITY (REPRODUCIBILITY, REPEATABILITY)

The extent to which a measurement produces the same result in the same situation

COMPONENTS OF ERROR

$$X_i = (T_i)B + a^* + \varepsilon_i + e_i$$

Where:

X_i = observed

T_i = true

B = proportional bias

a^* = constant bias

ε_i = random error ($\varepsilon_i = 0$)

e_i = bias in i^{th} subject ($e_i \neq 0$)

(underlying cause of differential misclassification)

OBSERVED VERSUS TRUE CLASSIFICATION

	True classification		
Observed classification	Low	Medium	High
Low	X		
Medium		X	
High			X

	True classification		
Observed classification	Low	Medium	High
Low	X	X	X
Medium	X	X	X
High	X	X	X

FUTURE WORK ON DIETARY ASSESSMENT IN RELATION TO FOOD SAFETY

- Harmonization of methods: e.g. EPIC, EUROFOODS

- New methods of dietary assessment and evaluation
  (e.g. IDA, PETRA, food photographs)

- New statistical techniques for combining results from several assessments to improve classification of subjects

- Improved understanding of differential misclassification, how it arises and how to handle it

PETRA

- Digital recording scales

    Place plate on scales
    Place food on plate
    Press black button

    weight recorded automatically

    voice recording of food description

- Master console

    Transcribes PETRA tape

    Finds each new entry

    Subtracts weights to find net weight of food

    Plays back recorded description of food

The Role of Databases:
The Example of a Food Plant Database

J. Gry, I. Søborg and I. Knudsen

Denmark

Introduction

In order to assess the novelty of food plants, whether they have been changed by traditional breeding techniques or by modern gene technology, the comparison can only be made if sufficient knowledge specifying the characteristics of the existing food plant products can be found.

The OECD suggested the introduction of the term "substantial equivalence" as a step in the overall evaluation of novel foods in its publication from 1993. Although no overall strategy to apply this tool is given yet, the discussion is going on worldwide, e.g. at this Workshop. We have suggested elsewhere that the first step in the evaluation procedure will involve the establishment of substantial equivalence based upon morphological equivalence, chemical equivalence, performance equivalence, and key substances equivalence.

This paper stresses the need for establishing an international plant database on toxic key substances, as well as key flavourings in our most common food plants.

The overall purpose is to establish knowledge which makes it possible to evaluate food plants, e.g. biotechnologically modified food plants or new exotic food plants, in order to establish whether their composition may constitute a health problem. The second purpose is to evaluate – supported by the database – whether modern food production, storage and preparation methods have a favourable or unfavourable influence on the constituents of the food plants and thereby on their health related and taste related capabilities. Thirdly, the database should support the counselling relating to the development of new food plants and to storage, preparation and cooking procedures with due respect to the health related and taste related importance of their chemical constituents.

The problem

The potentially adverse effects of many secondary plant metabolites, the so-called "inherent natural toxicants", in the human diet are now increasingly being recognized by many national and international organisations. Examples of such natural toxicants which may give rise to human intoxications are numerous, and include cyanogenic glycosides, pyrrolizidine alkaloids, furocoumarins, lectins and glycoalkaloids.

Dietary practices in line with current nutritional advice and recommendations (such as encouraging greater consumption of fruits and vegetables), and trends such as vegetarianism, use of health foods, and the developing interest in "functional foods" and "novel foods", including products from biotechnologically modified plants, may result in substantial increases in the human intakes of these natural toxicants. At present the consequences for human health are unclear, but it is widely agreed that these natural toxicants may present a greater risk for human health than, for instance, food additives and pesticide residues in the food. The lack of concrete evidence is especially due to the lack of critically evaluated data for use in the risk assessments, and consequently safety regulation, of these natural toxicants.

A number of the inherent natural toxicants are considered to play an important role in the plants' natural defence system, which offers protection against attack by fungi, insects or herbivores, or against the consequence of mechanical damage in the field or during the post-harvest storage. Genetic modification due to both traditional and modern biotechnology applied to the plants, followed by selection of new cultivars with enhanced natural resistance, often leads to substantial increases of these compounds or even to the presence of new compounds in the improved variety of the plant and the derived foodstuff.

There is considerable potential for the application of new technologies to improve the quality of major food crops across the European continent, and to increase the yield and extractability of "value-added" products. Therefore it is important to have access to reliable information on levels, mechanisms of action, and scopes for manipulating the levels of inherent toxicants.

The area of natural toxicant research has in the past been largely confined to the natural product chemist. Thus a great deal is known about the structures of the compounds involved, but the levels in the plants are generally far less well known and there is frequently little reliable data on the levels in the processed food as eaten, on the toxic effects of the individual substances, on any modifying effect of the food matrix, and on the significance of the latter for man. In addition, few studies have examined the importance of genetic, environmental or agronomic variables in modifying levels of natural toxicants.

There is thus a pressing need to develop and apply improved methods of analysis to determine levels of natural toxicants of crops, foods and derived products, and to make reliable estimates of intakes, both in the population as a whole, and in particular for risk sub-groups. Research is also required to determine the mechanisms of the toxic effect produced by these compounds and the mechanisms of the modifying, protective or synergistic effects of other dietary constituents. Risk assessments will need to be carried out on the basis of the above information. The extent to which levels of toxicants, identified as being a source of concern in the human diet, can be manipulated by plant breeding or by the application of modern biotechnology or improved processing techniques, also needs to be addressed.

The solution

Therefore a comprehensive and readily accessible information system containing data on the nature, levels, biological effects and significance of inherent plant toxins in the human diet is a prerequisite to direct and support these areas of research and regulatory activities. As data are scattered across the scientific literature and of very variable quality, it is vital that the compositional and toxicological data entered are critically assessed.

Today, there is no such internationally available information system covering food plants and their inherent toxicants and little information concerning flavourings in food plants.

The National Food Agency of Denmark realized back in 1988 the usefulness of such an information system for risk assessment, counselling and research concerning new food plants. The agency also realized the potential benefits for development of new food plants, for plant breeders and those importing fruits and vegetables, for establishments who store and prepare fruit and vegetables, as well as for producers of flavourings from natural source materials.

As of April 1994 the basic data for 200 food plants relating to natural inherent toxic compounds and flavourings are entered in the database. It is planned that the database should contain about 300 food plants presently used in Europe selected from a total of 600 to 700 food plants presently used as major food plants world-wide.

The database starts with the names and synonyms in twelve different European languages. (At the Oxford Workshop celery was taken as an example: see printout reproduced on the following pages.) The use (vegetable, fruit, herb, etc.) as well as the plant parts used (e.g. stalk, fruit, root) are given. For each of the plant parts used the nutritional constituents including amino acid composition and fatty acid composition are given, besides the toxic constituents and flavouring constituents. For each type of information the reference is given. So far the data included are mainly taken from internationally recognized handbooks and review articles in the field, considering their data to be of highest validity. The titles of the references are given in the last segment of the monograph. Besides this information unpublished data from the Centre for Food Research at the Royal Veterinary and Agricultural University, Copenhagen, and from the Danish Food Corporation DANISCO are entered. The database also includes very extended indices on chemical and botanical names. The database is elaborated in dBase 3+.

Originally the database project was financed by the National Food Agency, but due to lack of funding external sources were found and since 1992 the project has been financed by the Danish Research and Development Programme on Food Technology (FØTEK).

At present, information systems on natural food plant toxicants are being developed in Great Britain and Denmark, but there is a need to develop a common European system. Therefore we have submitted a proposal for the AAIR programme of the EU entitled "A European network to compile and evaluate data on natural food plant toxicants to assess risks to human health and to identify strategies to minimize such risks" (NETwork on TOXicants "NETTOX").

The objective of the proposed concerted action is to establish a European network of scientists dealing with inherent natural toxicants in food plants, to initiate and elaborate an information system containing critically evaluated compositional and toxicological data on natural toxicants, to initiate risk assessments on the most important European dietary plant toxicants based on information on human exposure and toxicological potential, and finally to study possible reduction of risks introduced by modern breeding and processing methods, while at the same time taking into consideration the agronomic, nutritional and organoleptic characters.

The application involves 15 countries, 33 individual scientists and four multinational food- producing companies. The European Commission has accepted the proposal for contract negotiations.

Celery

Apium graveolens

Names and synonyms

	Name	Synonym	Synonym
Species	Apium graveolens L.		
Family	Umbelliferae	Apiaceae	
DA	Selleri		
DE	Sellerie	Echter Sellerie	Zeller
EN	Celery	Celeriac	
ES	Apio		
FI	Selleri		
FR	Céleri		
GR	Selinon		
IS	Selleri		
IT	Sedano		
NL	Selderij		
NO	Selleri		
PT	Aipo		
SV	Selleri		

Used as

Vegetable

Plant parts used

1. Stalk, Leaf-
2. Root
3. Fruit

1. Plant part: Stalk, Leaf-

Nutritional Constituents		
	/100 g	References
Total carbohydrate	6.0 %	[51]
Sugars	1.2 %	[51]
Starch	0.1 %	[51]
Dietary fibers	dietary: 1.8 %	[51]
Vitamins	vitamin C: 7.1-14.2 mg/ 100 g	[51]
Minerals		
Protein 1)	0.8 %	[51]
Fat 2)	0.2 %	[51]

1) Amino Acid Composition	[51]
	mg/g N
Isoleucine	240
Leucine	430
Lysine	130
Methionine	110
Cystine	30
Phenylalanine	280
Tyrosine	80
Threonine	210
Tryptophane	70
Valine	300
Arginine	250
Histidine	90
Alanine	
Aspartic acid	
Glutamic acid	
Glycine	
Proline	
Serine	

2) Fatty Acid Composition						[51]
	g/100g fatty acid		g/100g fatty acid		g/100g fatty acid
C 4:0		C 14:1		C 18:2	53.8
C 6:0		C 15:1		C 18:3	
C 8:0		C 16:1	0.90	C 20:3	
C 10:0		C 17:1		C 20:4	
C 12:0		C 18:1	20.6	C 20:5	
C 14:0	0.90	C 20:1		C 22:5	
C 15:0		C 22:1		C 22:6	
C 16:0	25.1	Others		Others	
C 17:0					
C 18:0	2.69				
C 20:0					
C 22:0					
Others					
Sum	28.7	Sum	21.5	Sum	53.8

1. Plant part: Stalk, Leaf-

Toxic Constituents			
Groups	Substances	Amounts in mg/kg	References
Coumarins	Bergapten	see 5-Methoxypsoralen	
	5,8-Dimethoxypsoralen	0-1.22	[179]
	Furanocoumarin	= furocoumarin	
	Isopimpinellin	see 5,8-Dimethoxypsoralen	
	Linear furocoumarins	see Psoralens	
	5-Methoxypsoralen	0.33-1.45	[179]
	8-Methoxypsoralen	0.37-1.83	[179]
	5-Methoxypsoralen	0.53-2.87	[198]
	5-Methoxypsoralen	up to 8.55 (diseased)	[198]
	8-Methoxypsoralen	0.86-3.81	[198]
	8-Methoxypsoralen	up to 21.35 (diseased)	[198]
	Psoralen	present	[179]
	Psoralen	<0.06-1.98	[198]
	Psoralen	up to 14.14 (diseased)	[198]
	Psoralens	up to 24 totally	[157]
	Psoralens	normally <1.3	[197]
	Psoralens	18 in phototoxic brand	[166]
	Psoralens	1.4-8.4	[198]
	Psoralens	up to 43.81 (diseased)	[198]
	Xanthotoxin	see 8-Methoxypsoralen	
Lectins	Lectins	Reported	[154]
Others	Apiole	see Parsley apiole	
	Cholinesterase inhibitor		[121]
	Myristicin	0.33	[179]

1. Plant part: Stalk, Leaf-

Flavouring Constituents			
Groups	Substances	Amounts in mg/kg	References
Essential Oils - Continued	Hexanal	0.47	[179]
	Hexane		[179]
	1-Hexanol	0.2	[179]
	cis-3-Hexen-1-ol	4.5	[179]
	trans-2-Hexen-1-ol	0.2	[179]
	cis-3-Hexenyl 2-oxopropanoate		[179]
	cis-3-Hexenyl acetate	0.04	[179]
	alpha-Humulene		[179]
	beta-Humulene		[179]
	4-Hydroxydecanoic acid lactone		[179]
	alpha-Ionone	0.2	[179]
	Isoamyl alcohol	see 3-Methyl-1-butanol	
	1-Isobutylidenephthalide	0.001	[179]
	Isobutyric acid	see 2-Methylpropanoic acid	
	Isopimpinellin	see 5,8-Dimethoxypsoralen	
	1-Isopropenyl-4-methylbenzene	0.12	[179]
	1-Isopropyl-4-methylbenzene	0.18-0.3	[179]
	Isopropylbenzene		[179]
	3-Isovalidenephthalide	0.001	[179]
	Ligustilide	see 3-Butylidene-4,5-dihydrophthalide	
	Limonene	214	[179]
	cis-Limonene oxide (unkn.str.)	1.1	[179]
	trans-Limonene oxide (unkn.str.)	0.1-0.8	[179]
	Linalool		[179]
	Linalyl acetate		[179]
	Linoleic acid	see cis-9,cis-12-Octadecadienoic acid	

2. Plant part: Root

Nutritional Constituents		
	/100 g	References
Total carbohydrate	8.3 %	[51]
Sugars	1.8 %	[51]
Starch	0.37 %	[51]
Dietary fibers	dietary: 4.2 %	[51]
Vitamins	beta-Carotene: 30 microg./100 g	[51]
Minerals		
Protein 1)	1.8 %	[51]
Fat 2)	0.3 %	[51]

1) Amino Acid Composition	[51]
	mg/g N
Isoleucine	190
Leucine	300
Lysine	300
Methionine	74
Cystine	13
Phenylalanine	190
Tyrosine	99
Threonine	180
Tryptophane	47
Valine	290
Arginine	180
Histidine	94
Alanine	340
Aspartic acid	670
Glutamic acid	1150
Glycine	190
Proline	160
Serine	200

2) Fatty Acid Composition						[51]
	g/100g fatty acid		g/100g fatty acid		g/100g fatty acid
C 4:0		C 14:1		C 18:2	59.2
C 6:0		C 15:1		C 18:3	6.58
C 8:0		C 16:1		C 20:3	
C 10:0		C 17:1		C 20:4	0
C 12:0		C 18:1	4.74	C 20:5	
C 14:0		C 20:1		C 22:5	
C 15:0		C 22:1		C 22:6	
C 16:0	23.7	Others	0.52	Others	
C 17:0					
C 18:0	1.32				
C 20:0					
C 22:0					
Others	3.88				
Sum	28.9	Sum	5.26	Sum	65.78

2. Plant part: Root

Toxic Constituents			
Groups	Substances	Amounts in mg/kg	References
Coumarins	Bergapten	see 5-Methoxypsoralen	
	5,8-Dimethoxypsoralen	1.7-12.6	[186]
	Isopimpinellin	see 5,8-Dimethoxypsoralen	
	Linear furocoumarins	see Psoralens	
	5-Methoxypsoralen	1.5-31.5	[186]
	8-Methoxypsoralen	1.6-10.4	[186]
	Psoralen	0.1-6.3	[186]
	Psoralens	total of phototoxic 4.5-46.7	[186]
	Psoralens	equiv. to 100 8-MOP found	[199]
	Psoralens	1.7-16.7 in edible part	[186]
	Psoralens, phototoxic	up to 58.6 in peel	[186]
	Xanthotoxin	see 8-Methoxypsoralen	
Others	Apiin		[3] [12]
	Cholinesterase inhibitor		[121]
	Toxic polyacetylen compounds		[3]

3. Plant part: Fruit

Toxic Constituents

Groups	Substances	Amounts in mg/kg	References
Coumarins	Bergapten	see 5-Methoxypsoralen	
	5,8-Dimethoxypsoralen	approx. 0.5	[180]
	8-Hydroxy-5-methoxypsoralen		[179]
	7-Hydroxycoumarin	present	[179]
	Isopimpinellin	see 5,8-Dimethoxypsoralen	
	Linear furocoumarins	see Psoralens	
	5-Methoxypsoralen	2.3-16.93	[180]
	Umbelliferone	see 7-Hydroxycoumarin	
Others	Cholinesterase inhibitor		[121]
	Myristicin		[121]
	Myristicin	1800 of essential oil	[179]

3. Plant part: Fruit

Flavouring Constituents			
Groups	Substances	Amounts in mg/kg	References
Essential Oils		1.5-2.5 % of dry fruit	[6]
		2-3 % of dry fruit	[3]
		2.5-3 % of dry fruit	[20]
		Conc. where not otherwise specified mg/kg ess. oil	
	4-Allyl-2-methoxyphenol		[179]
	6-Allyl-4-methoxy-1,3-benzodioxole	see Myristicin	
	Bergapten	see 5-Methoxypsoralen	
	3-Butyl-4,5-dihydrophthalide	38000-91000	[179]
	3-Butylidene-4,5-dihydrophthalide	15000-45000	[179]
	3-Butylidenetetrahydrophthalide (unkn.str)		[179]
	3-Butylphthalide	9000-40000	[179]
	Butylphthalide (unkn.str.)	25600	[179]
	3-Butyltetrahydrophthalide		[179]
	Camphene	trace-400	[179]
	3-Carene	trace-300	[179]
	Carvone	900-2000	[179]
	beta-Caryophyllene	1000-14000	[179]
	Caryophyllene oxide (unkn.str.)	3000-5500	[179]
	Cinnamaldehyde	1500	[179]
	p-Cymene	see 1-Isopropyl-4-methylbenzene	
	Cymol	see 1-Isopropyl-4-methylbenzene	
	3a,4-Dihydro-3-isobutylidene-phthalide	0.7	[179]
	3a,4-Dihydro-3-isovalidenephthalide	0.2	[179]
	6,7-Dihydro-8-hydroxy-7-isopropenyl-psoralen		[179]
	5,8-Dimethoxypsoralen		[179]

References

Numbers	Titles
166	Beier, R.C. Natural Pesticides and Bioactive Components in Foods Rev. Environ. Contam. Toxicol. 1990. vol. 113. p. 47-137 Springer-Verlag New York Inc.
179	Maarse, H. and Visscher, C.A. Editors Volatile Compounds in Food, 6.th Edition, Supplement 1 TNO Biotechnology and Chemistry Institute, AJ Zeist, The Netherlands, 1990.
180	Ceska, O., Chaudhary, S.K., Warrington, P.J. and Ashwood-Smith, M.J. Photoactive Furocoumarins in Fruits of Some Umbellifers Phytochemistry, 26 (1), 1987, p. 165-169
186	Baumann, U., Dick, R. and Zimmerli, B. Orientierende Untersuchung zum Vorkommen von Furocoumarinen in pflanzlichen Lebensmitteln und Kosmetika. Mitt. Gebiete Lebensm. Hyg. 1988, 79, p. 112.
197	Beier, R.C., Ivie, G.W., Oertli, E.H., and Holt, D.L. HPLC Analysis of Linear Furocoumarins (Psoralens) in Healthy Celery (Apium graveolens) Food Chem. Toxic., 1983, 21 (2), p. 163-165.
198	Chaudhary, S.K., Ceska, O., Warrington P.J., and Ashwood-Smith, M.J. Increased Furocoumarin Content of Celery during Storage J. Agric. Food Chem., 1985, 33, p. 1153-1157.
199	Ljunggren, B. Severe Phototoxic Burn Following Celery Ingestion Arch. Dermatol., 1990, 126, p. 1334-1336.

The Use of *in vivo* and *in vitro* Models in the Testing of Microorganisms

Bodil Lund Jacobsen

Institute of Toxicology
National Food Agency of Denmark

Introduction

New biotechniques such as genetic engineering and cell fusion will change our food supply in the years to come. These changes raise a number of questions in relation to impact on food safety and control.

Genetically modified microorganisms will contribute both indirectly and directly to food production. Indirectly, microorganisms will be used for production of food additives and enzymes. Directly, they may produce single cell proteins, beer, cheese and yoghurt.

Fifteen to twenty years ago, genetic engineering in bacteria led to a number of specific questions: Could there be unexpected or possible biological side effects due to inserted genes? Could genetic changes result in altered ability to survive and colonize the human gut? What about the transfer of introduced genes to other microorganisms? How was it possible to elucidate the fate and effect of genetically modified microorganisms (GMOs)?

At the Institute of Toxicology, risk assessments of chemicals and the use of laboratory animals in toxicology testing were already well established disciplines. Our aim was to extend the traditional toxicology to include risk assessment and testing of GMOs.

***In vivo* and *in vitro* models**

In order to evaluate the fate and effect of GMOs we have established different *in vivo* and *in vitro* models of the mammalian gut. The mammalian gut was chosen because it is a likely route of exposure in connection with the release of GMOs, including intake of modified food.

Table 1 presents the mammalian intestinal models, ranging from conventional *in vivo* models to *in vitro* models. The different models show different levels of colonization resistance. Colonization resistance is the ability of a microflora to resist the colonization of new microorganisms (Van der Waiij et al., 1971). In practice the presence of a normal intestinal flora of conventional animals, including man, will often result in the elimination of the introduced bacteria. A test microorganism with an antibiotic resistance marker can be followed analyzing faecal samples by the simple plate spread method. In the conventional rat, mouse and minipig the test microorganism *Escherichia coli* is eliminated from faecal samples within six days.

The use of antibiotics results in the disturbance of the normal protective flora and allows for the introduction of new bacteria. Norfloxacin is an antibiotic that selectively eliminates Enterobacteriacea from the gastrointestinal flora (Van der Waiij et al., 1989). The use of norfloxacin creates a hole in the protective barrier that allows for colonization with newly introduced *Escherichia coli*. The treatment of mice with streptomycin resulting in a disturbed microflora, and hence reduced colonizations resistance, has also been used in the investigation of different *E. coli* K12 strains (Cohen et al., 1979). Compared to the streptomycin model, the norfloxacin model has a great advantage. Norfloxacin need not to be given to the animals continuously and does not exert a constant selective pressure on the test bacteria.

Using specific *E. coli* strains, a norfloxacin treated pig and a two-stage chemostat model of the intestinal microflora of the norfloxacin treated pig made it possible to study the colonization ability of two closely related *E. coli* strains. None of the strains colonized a conventional minipig or the corresponding *in vitro* model of an intact porcine flora. The results indicated that it would be possible to construct and use an *in vitro* model of the mammalian intestine in order to distinguish between strains of different colonization abilities (Nielsen and Schlundt 1992).

An even further reduction in colonization resistance is seen in the germ-free rat, the definition of germ-free life being "free from any other *detectable* form of life" (Gustafsson, 1984). The microbial status of germ-free animals is achieved and maintained using isolators. The germ-free rats are housed in a closed sterile plastic bubble, in which a suitable and defined environment is maintained. The work of keeping the rats germ-free is hard and tedious – however, the experimental advantages make up for it. The germ-free rats provide a defined system with intact biological parameters. This allows for a free choice in the introduction of microorganisms. Introducing a test microorganism into the germ-free rat often results in long term colonization in high concentrations, which is very important in the study of processes like gene transfer.

The use of models in the study of survival/colonization and gene transfer

Much of our research using germ-free rats is related to the concept of biological containment. The concept of biological containment basically involves two aspects: survival of the microorganisms and gene transfer. Biological containment is very important when considering environmental releases of GMOs. One would like the modified microorganism to live and perform, but not to survive forever. With this reasoning in mind, S. Molin and co-workers proposed a containment principle, which relies on imposing a growth disadvantage in the released populations rather than on debilitation of the individual cell. A gene *hok*, coding for a small protein lethal to the cell, is activated at random by the *E. coli fim* A promoter, thereby resulting in killing a constant fraction of the released microorganisms per unit time (Molin et al., 1987). The constructions have been tested *in vitro* in simple test tubes. Our aim was to investigate the fate of a wild type *E. coli* containing a plasmid with the suicide gene *hok* in the intestine *in vivo*.

The experimental design in our investigation was based upon the effect of the lethal gene on the rate of decline/exclusion of a secondary invader in the gut. We wanted to create a situation of competition between two closely related bacteria, leading to the possible exclusion of the newly introduced strain. This is a situation which is most likely to occur in nature. Initially we dosed wild type *E. coli* p.o. with a single high dose intragastrically, and shortly afterward we found a high stable concentration of E. coli in faecal samples resembling the resident population. At day 0 the genetically modified bacteria, E. coli with the hok gene was introduced, and in competition with the residents this secondary strain declined. This was to be expected, but compared to a similar experiment, where the secondary invader did not carry the hok gene, we could see a difference. Carrying out regression analysis we were able to compute and use T_{90} values as a measure of decline, T_{90} being the time used for a 90 per cent reduction of the bacterial concentration. The mean elimination time was 2.8 days for E. coli with the hok gene in contrast to 5.3 days for the E. coli without the hok gene (Jacobsen et al., 1993).

Apart from the study of survival and colonization, the germ-free rats have also been used for the study of the transfer of genetic material from one microorganism to another. We have studied a containment principle inhibiting gene transfer in the test microorganism E. coli. The same test strategy used for E. coli have also been used for microorganisms relevant for food. Gnotobiotic rats have been used in the study of the conjugal transfer of plasmid DNA between Lactococcus lactis strains and the distribution of transconjugants in the intestinal tract. In the study we were able to measure the conjugal transfer of plasmid pAMß1 between strains of Lactococcus lactis subsp. lactis. Germ-free rats were dosed intragastrically with the recipient strain and the donor strain carrying pAMß1. In faecal samples from the dosed gnotobiotic rats, transconjugants were observed soon after dosing colonizing the intestine. At the end of the experiment, the animals were necropsied and samples from duodenum, jejunum, caecum and colon were cultured for the presence of donor, recipient and transconjugants. The concentration of transconjugants was approximately 10^4 c.f.u./g throughout the intestine, whereas the concentration of recipients increased from 10^4 -10^5 c.f.u./g in the jejunum to 10^8 -10^9 c.f.u./g in caecum and colon (Schlundt el al., 1994).

All of these studies were based on the use of selective antibiotic resistance markers. The Advisory Committee on Novel Foods and Processes has recently produced a report on the use of antibiotic resistance markers in genetically modified food organisms. In the report the committee is adopting the strategy that genetically modified food microorganisms which are intended to be ingested live should not contain antibiotic resistance markers. An example of a non-selectable marker is the very elegant construction made in Lactococcus lactis by Dr C. Hertel resulting in a silent mutation in a proteinase gene. This genetic modification may be used as an marker without disturbing the phenotype of the microorganism (Hertel et al., 1992). At present we have, in co-operation with universities in Stuttgart and Munich, concluded experiments in which we have tested Lactococcus lactis with the plasmid pLMP1 carrying this silent mutation using gnotobiotic rats. Besides testing the transfer of pLMP1 in comparison with the plasmid pAMß1, we have also used DNA techniques for the detection of the genetically modified microorganism (manuscript in preparation).

Finally, I would like to summarize concerning the testing of microorganisms in general. It is very difficult to use *in vivo* or *in vitro* models to assess the pathogenicity of GMOs for humans, but we may try. The extrapolation from animal to man can be reduced by using an human intestinal flora associated rat or *in vitro* models based on the human microflora. The experience gained from the use of advanced *in vivo* and *in vitro* models of the mammalian gut might, combined with experience from the work with established guidelines (as an example, the guidelines for testing of microbial plant protection products) be useful in the design of guidelines for the testing of microorganisms in food.

Table 1
Mammalian Intestinal Models

	Rat	Mouse	Pig	Human
Conventional	+	+	+	
Norfloxacin treated	+	+	+	-
Streptomycin treated	+	+	-	-
Germ-free	+	-	-	*)
2-stage chemostat	+		+	+

+ = Model established

*) = Human Faecal Flora Associated, a gnotobiotic rat to be established in 1995.

Table 2
Factors Limiting Biological Containment

1. The ability of a genetic modified organism to survive and disseminate in the environment.

2. Transfer of genetic material to other organisms in the environment.

Note: The degree of biological containment depends on an evaluation of both the host and the vector.

References

Cohen, P.S., Pilsucki, R.W., Myhal, M.L., Rosen, C.A., Laux, D.C. and Cabelli, V.J. (1979) Colonization potentials of male and female *E. coli* K12 strains, *E. coli* B and human fecal *E. coli* strains in the mouse GI tract. *Recomb. DNA Tech. Bull.* 2:106-113.

Gustafsson, B.E. (1984) Introduction. The germ-free animal: its potential and its problems. In: Coates M.E. and Gustafsson, B.E. (eds.) *The germ-free animal in biomedical research*. Laboratory Animal Handbooks No. 9. Laboratory Animals Ltd., London.

Hertel, C., Wolfgang, L. and Schleifer, K.H. (1992) Introduction of silent mutations in a proteinase gene of *Lactococcus lactis* as a useful marker for monitoring studies. *System. Appl. Microbiol.* 15:447-452.

Jacobsen, B.L., Schlundt, J. and Fischer, G. (1993). Study of a conditional suicide system for biological containment of bacteria in germ-free rats. *Microbial Ecology in Health and Disease* 6:109-118.

Molin, S., Klemm, P., Poulsen, L.K., Biehl, H., Gerdes, K. and Andersson, P. (1987) Conditional suicide system for containment of bacteria and plasmids. *Bio/Technology* 5:1315-1318.

Nielsen, E.M. and Schlundt, J. (1992) Use of norfloxacin to study colonization ability of *Escherichia coli in vivo* and *in vitro* models of the porcine gut. *Antimicrobial Agents and Chemotherapy* 36:401-407.

Schlundt, J., Saadbye, P., Lohmann, B., Jacobsen, B.L. and Nielsen, E.M. (1994) Conjugal transfer of plasmid DNA between *Lactococcus lactis* strains and distribution of transconjugants in the digestive tract of gnotobiotic rats.

van der Waiij, D., Berghuis-de Vries, J.M. and Lekkerkerk-van der Wees, J.E.C. (1971) Colonization resistance of the digestive tract in conventional and antibiotic-treated mice. *Journal of Hygiene* 69:405-411.

van der Waiij, L.A., Messerschmidt, O. and van der Waiij, D. (1989) A norfloxaxin dose finding study for the selective decontamination of the digestive tract in pigs. *Epidemiol. Infect.* 102, 93-103.

The Application of Human-type Diets in Rodent Feeding Studies for the Safety Evaluation of Novel Foods

A.C. Huggett, M. Marchesini, I. Perrin, B. Schilter, J.C. Tschantz, A. Donnet,
P. Morgenthaler, G. Sunahara and H-P. Würzner

Department of Quality and Safety Assurance
Nestec Ltd. Research Centre
Switzerland

Summary

Traditional food safety evaluation studies were designed for additives and other components consumed in small quantities and comprising an insignificant proportion of the diet. The development of novel foods which may comprise a more substantial part of the diet, poses several problems with regard to their safety evaluation by conventional testing procedures such as the subchronic rodent feeding study in rodents. These may result from nutritional disturbances caused by the addition of large quantities of test material to a basal rodent diet. Additionally, in the case of the safety assessment of novel processes, the significance of the effects of the novel processing/treatment procedures on non-human diets may be questionable. The application of human-type diets, with interchangeable macroconstituents, adapted for the nutritional needs of rodents may overcome some of these problems. A 90-day subchronic feeding study in rats was used to compare the effects of a human-type diet based on industrial dried and pre-cooked ingredients (carrots, potatoes, green beans, couscous, lentils and granulated meat) with a conventional semi-synthetic rodent diet. Various diagnostic toxicological parameters were examined, including clinical chemistry, haematology, histology, immunological markers, and xenobiotic metabolizing activities. The human-type diet was well accepted and adequate for the normal nutrition and development of the rodents. Minor differences in certain parameters were detected, most likely reflecting the different compositions of the major dietary components. However, all of these were within in-house established normal values. No evidence of overt toxicity was detected, although the human-type diet provoked a simple hyperplasia of the urinary bladder epithelium in male rats. Although the toxicological significance of this finding is unclear, it does not pose a problem for subchronic studies. In conclusion the use of modified basal diets in toxicological studies may provide a practical approach for the safety evaluation of novel foods.

Introduction

Traditional food safety evaluation procedures have been designed for components consumed in small quantities and comprising an insignificant portion of the diet. The introduction of novel foods and processes poses new challenges for food toxicologists and regulators, and there is a need for the development of new conceptual tools for food safety assessment. The objective of this study is to investigate the feasibility of a new approach applicable to the safety evaluation of two specific groups of novel foods: (a) those produced using a novel process; and (b) those which comprise a substantial part of the diet (macrocomponents).

In those cases where it is deemed necessary to perform a subchronic feeding study in order to investigate the safety of a novel food process or treatment, the choice of test material can be perplexing, especially when the novel process is intended for application to a multitude of diverse food components or whole foods. One strategy is to test conventional rodent diets which have been subjected to the novel process. However, this approach may be questionable due to the unrepresentative composition of the rodent diets compared to the typical human diet. This problem may be resolved by the use of rodent-adapted diets which more closely reflect the diversity of constituents of the normal human diet.

The development of novel foods which comprise a substantial part of the diet pose several problems with regard to their safety evaluation by conventional testing procedures. For example, apparent toxic effects may result from nutritional imbalances caused by the addition of large quantities of test material to the basal rodent diet rather than from the inherent toxicity of the novel food. Feeding studies to assess the safety of macrocomponents is complicated, since the use of NOAELS may not be applicable and thus it is impossible to obtain sufficiently large safety factors to assure the reasonable safety of the product in humans. In order to overcome this, it is necessary to improve the sensitivity and diagnostic capabilities of the traditional subchronic feeding study. Two complimentary strategies can be undertaken to achieve this. The first is the use of nutritional balanced diets with interchangeable macroconstituents, which allows a maximization of the dose of test component that can be incorporated. The second strategy is to identify early sensitive markers of potential inherent toxicity. Some of these markers may then be applicable in controlled confirmatory studies in humans of the macrocomponent in question.

In order to investigate the utility of these approaches, we have investigated the application of human-type diets, with interchangeable macroconstituents adapted to meet the nutritional needs of rodents, in a conventional rodent subchronic feeding study. The further development of this approach will be the validation and incorporation of parameters in toxicological studies which serve as sensitive early predictive and diagnostic markers of cellular and organ toxicity.

Materials and methods

Animals and animal care

Male and female Sprague-Dawley rats obtained from Iffa Credo S.A. (L'Arbresle, France) were housed individually throughout the study period. The animals underwent an 11-day adaptation period with the reference diet prior to being placed on the experimental diets for 13 weeks. They were randomized according to body weight into the two different treatment groups (reference diet, human-type diet) of 10 animals/sex 1 wk before the start of the study. At the initiation of treatment (=day 0) the animals were about 4-5 wk old, with mean body weights of 134 g (males) and 126 g (females). Diets and tap water were available *ad libitum*.

Diets

The reference (control) diet was modified AIN-76 (American Institute of Nutrition, 1977), a semi-synthetic diet (**Table 1**). The basis of the test diet was an industrial dry mix of pre-cooked meat, dehydrated mashed potatoes, lyophilized green beans, carrots, lentils and couscous (**Table 2**). The ingredients were mixed in such a ratio that the macronutrients in the finished diet approximated those of the reference diet (**Figure 1**). The human-type diet was supplemented with vitamins, minerals, choline bitartrate and inositol to meet the nutritional requirements of the rat.

Observations and analyses

The animals were observed daily for condition and behaviour, while body weights, water consumption and food intake were measured weekly. At the end of the experimental period, the animals were fasted (20-22 hr), anaesthetized with Pentobarbital (60 mg/kg body weight, i.p.) and sacrificed by exsanguination from the abdominal aorta.

Haematology and clinical chemistry

Blood samples collected from the abdominal aorta were analysed for total red and white blood cell counts; haematocrit; haemoglobin content; platelets; reticulocytes (Cellanalyser CA 480, Medonic Servotec, Switzerland); differential white blood cell counts (microscopic examination of stained blood smears); and prothrombin time (Micro Coagulometer, Greiner, Switzerland). The blood clinical chemistry parameters examined were: total bilirubin; glucose; alkaline phosphatase activity (ALP); aspartate aminotransferase activity (ASAT); alanine aminotransferase activity (ALAT); lactate dehydrogenase activity (LDH); 5'-nucleotidase activity (5-NU); -glutamyl transferase activity (-GT); amylase; albumin; calcium; creatinine; urea (BUN); phosphate; iron; magnesium; total cholesterol; free fatty acids; triglycerides; phospholipids; sodium; potassium; chloride; total protein; protein electrophoresis; (COBAS Bio, Roche Diagnostics, Switzerland); lipoproteins (Tschantz and Sunahara, 1993); protein electrophoretic profile (Beckman Microzone, Beckman, Nyon, Switzerland).

Pathology

All tissues were carefully examined macroscopically. The liver, kidneys, spleen, heart, adrenals, testes, thymus, pancreas and brain were weighed and organ-to-body and organ-to-brain weights were calculated. Samples of all tissues were removed for microscopic histological evaluation.

FACs analysis of cell surface markers

Blood collected into potassium-EDTA was passed over Ficoll Hypaque (Sigma, St. Louis, USA). Cells collected at the interface were washed and finally re-suspended in a 1/100 dilution of normal serum in phosphate buffered saline (pH 7.4). Direct immunofluorescence labelling (1 hr at 4°C in the dark), to identify CD3, CD4, CD8 and Major Histocompatibility Complex Class II antigen (MHC-II), was performed using FITC-conjugated monoclonal antibodies 1F4, W3/25, OX8 and OX6 respectively (Serotec, Oxford, England). FITC-conjugated mouse IgG1 protein (Becton Dickinson) served as the isotype control. After labelling, cells were washed and then fixed for one hr in 1 per cent paraformaldehyde prior to re-suspension in sheath fluid (Becton Dickinson). Flow cytometric analysis was performed using a FACScan (Becton Dickinson).

Liver Xenobiotic Metabolic Activity

Samples of fresh liver tissue were taken for preparation of microsomal and S9 fractions according to Marow and Ames, 1983. Liver microsomes were used for the measurement of various xenobiotic metabolizing activities: ethoxycoumarin O-deethylase (Greenlee and Poland, 1978), ethoxyresorufin O-deethylase (e) and pentoxyresorufin O-deethylase (PROD) according to Burke et al., (1985); and erythromycin demethylase according to the method of Wrighton et al., (1985). The ability of the liver S9 fraction to activate (2-amino-3,8-dimethylimidazo[4,5-]quinoxaline) MeIQx to mutagenic metabolites was assessed in the Ames test (Marow and Ames; 1983).

Results

All animals survived the 13-week feeding period and there were no treatment-related alterations in the appearance or behaviour of the animals. The animals fed the human-type diet showed normal growth (**Figure 2**) and correspondingly similar terminal body weights were observed at autopsy. The food consumption, particularly for males fed this diet, was increased compared to animals fed the reference diet and this was paralleled by a slightly increased water consumption (Figure 2).

There were few statistically significant treatment-related differences in haematological and clinical chemistry parameters in animals fed the different diets (**Table 3**). Slightly, but significantly, lower values for haemoglobin concentration and mean platelet volume were found in both sexes fed the test diet. Differences in clinical chemistry values observed in both sexes were limited to a decreased bilirubin and 5'-nucleotidase activity in animals fed the human-type diet. In addition, male animals fed this diet demonstrated increases in amylase, potassium and chlorides, while decreases was observed for total cholesterol, phospholipids, free fatty acids and iron. Cholesterol was decreased in both HDL and LDL fractions and the overall LDL/HDL ratio was also decreased. Serum protein electrophoresis showed an increase in the -globulin fraction in males fed the human-type diet.

Organ weights of animals fed the human-type diet did not show any significant differences from those fed the reference diet with the exception of the liver weight of male animals, which was increased in absolute terms and also relative to both body and brain weight (Table 3). In females the increase in liver weight was only observed when expressed relative to body weight. In both sexes the weight of the kidneys was increased relative to body weight in animals fed the human-type diet, and the thymus weight of females was decreased in absolute terms and relative to brain weight. Gross examination at autopsy did not reveal any treatment-related changes.

In the liver, a decreased prominence of cytoplasmic vacuolation of periportal hepatocytes was observed in animals of both sexes fed the human diet as compared to controls, and the appearance of hepatocellular "ground-glass" cytoplasm was more apparent in males fed the human diet (**Table 4**). In these latter animals large globular or rod-shaped inclusions were observed in the cytoplasm of cells of single proximal convoluted tubules in the kidney. They stained orange to yellow with PAS and deeply red with Mallory Heidenhain. Both the incidence and severity of spontaneous corticomedullary mineralization, a very frequent finding in female laboratory rats, were decreased in females on human diet. Simple urothelial hyperplasia of the urinary bladder was observed in 9 males and 2 females fed the human diet. This was manifested by a slight increase in the number of epithelial cell layers and a marked increase in the number of nuclei per surface unit. Although haemosiderin stored in red-pulp macrophages was observed in most rat spleens, it tended to be more prominent in both males and females on human diet. Deposits per cell were larger and the incidence of macrophages containing haemosiderin was increased. No other histological changes related to diet were observed in the other tissues examined.

There were no statistically significant changes in the proportion of CD3 (T-lymphocytes), CD4 (T-helper cells, macrophages) or CD8 (T-suppressor cells, natural killer cells) positive cells in the blood from treated animals compared to controls (**Figure 3**). In addition, the proportion of cells expressing MHC-II, a marker for activated T cells and monocytes, was similar in animals fed the different diets.

The activity of certain key phase I liver xenobiotic-metabolizing enzymes (cytochrome P450 1A, P450 IIB, P450 IIIA families) was similar in animals fed either of the diets (**Figure 4**). In addition the ability of liver S9 fractions to activate the food mutagen MeIQx to mutagenic metabolites was comparable for the two groups although samples prepared from male animals were less active than those from females (Figure 4).

Discussion

The experimental human-type diet was well accepted by the animals and was adequate for their normal development and behaviour in the absence of adverse effects. The slightly reduced body weight evolution of animals fed the human-type diet in comparison with the reference rodent diet was largely compensated by the increased food intake. This finding is most likely due to the slightly reduced caloric density of the human diet and the slight, but nutritionally relevant difference in composition between the two diets, particularly the higher fat and lower moisture content of the reference AIN-76 diet.

A summary of treatment-related findings is provided in Tables 3 and 4. With the exception of the effects of the human-type diet on bladder epithelial histology, all observations remained within in-house established normal limits for the strain of rat used in this study. The effects observed most likely reflect a metabolic adaptation to the different composition of the major dietary proteins and lipids present in the human-type diet compared to the reference diet.

The reduced haemoglobin and serum iron, which were accompanied by a slightly increased haemosiderin storage in splenic macrophages suggest that in animals fed the human-type diet iron tended to be preferentially stored in the spleen rather than incorporated into haemoglobin or distributed to the tissues. Neither qualitative morphological evaluation nor an investigation of blood immunological parameters revealed an equivalent for the decreased thymus weight recorded in females on human diet, which is most likely due to the incomplete removal of adherent tissue at autopsy.

There were some differential effects of the human-type diet on liver histology and diagnostic blood parameters compared to the reference diet. In rats of both sexes fed the test diet, physiological hepatocellular lipid storage was somewhat decreased. Cytoplasmic changes indicating hypertrophy of smooth endoplasmic reticulum and increased glycogen accumulation (Jones et al., 1985) were restricted to males, and probably account for the increased liver weight. Alterations in blood biochemical parameters were found predominantly in males. These were indicative of changes in the metabolism of carbohydrates (increased serum amylase), proteins (decreased 5'-NU) and lipids (decreased total cholesterol, lipoproteins, phospholipids and free fatty acids, increased -globulin).

In males fed the human-type diet, cytoplasmic inclusions were observed in the proximal convoluted tubules of the kidney. Although quite large, they appeared to be biologically inert, causing neither degeneration or hyperplasia nor tubular casts. Their probable aetiology may be as a result of an increased filtration of small soluble dietary proteins through the glomerular basement membrane and their accumulation in tubular cells subsequent to their reabsorption. As these inclusions were in most cases restricted to single tubules, they are unlikely to account for the increased kidney weight relative to body weight observed in animals fed the human-type diet, which appears to be a physiological adaptation to the diet. The incidence and severity of renal corticomedullary mineralization, a common finding in female laboratory rats (Ritskes-Hoitinga and Beynen, 1992), was decreased in females fed the test diet.

Simple hyperplasia of the urinary bladder epithelium with a diffuse distribution pattern was observed mainly in males fed the human-type diet. There was no evidence of inflammation or mechanical damage which could cause hyperplasia, and the cause of this effect is presently unknown. The toxicological relevance of this finding is not clear since the present experiment does not allow conclusions as to reversibility or long-term evolution of the urothelial hyperplasia. Interestingly, however, similar findings were observed in a recent subchronic feeding study of rats with human-type diets subjected to different cooking regimens (Jonkers and Til, 1993). Nevertheless, this finding does not pose a problem for subchronic studies and so does not preclude the use of the human-type diet in the safety evaluation of novel foods.

The lack of test diet-related effects on the activity of several key phase I xenobiotic metabolizing enzymes indicates that the potential activation/detoxification of dietary components or contaminants would be similar in animals fed the human-type diet compared to rodent diets currently used in toxicity testing. This is further supported by the similar mutagenic activation potency (MeIQx) of liver S9 fractions from animals fed the test and reference diets.

The objective of this study was to examine the viability of using a human-type diet in subchronic rodent toxicology studies. This type of toxicity study is a standard for the safety evaluation of food components such as additives. However, it requires modifications if it is to be meaningfully applied to the safety evaluation of certain classes of novel foods. The use of a human-type diet with interchangeable macroconstituents is a potential strategy for overcoming some of the issues associated with the safety assessment of these foods. The potential application of this strategy is dependent upon several criteria: 1) the human-type diet must satisfy the nutritional requirements of the rat; 2) the basic constituents of the diet must be standardised and subject to minimal variation; 3) the human-type diet must be stable over the duration of a study; 4) the diet must be acceptable to rodents and produce no adverse effects.

The human-type diet used in the present study adequately satisfies these criteria. The use of human diets in toxicological studies in rats was previously reported by Alink et al., 1989). However, in that study the human diet was not completely balanced to meet the nutritional requirements of the rat and differed markedly from the conventional rodent diet with regard to macronutrient content and caloric value. Consequently, these discrepancies led to differences in certain important diagnostic parameters demonstrating the importance of the prevention of nutritional imbalances in toxicological studies.

There are two potential applications of such an approach with regard to the safety evaluation of novel foods: 1) safety evaluation of novel processes; 2) safety evaluation of macroconstituents (e.g. fat replacers, transgenic plants). The concept of applying a human-type diet for the evaluation of the potential toxicological effects of food processes has recently been successfully demonstrated in a subchronic feeding study to confirm the safety of microwave cooking (Jonker and Til, 1993). Such a diet was used in order that the effects of this treatment/process on ingredients commonly used in human foods could be assessed. This strategy is potentially applicable to the testing of novel processes which may be applied to a variety of different food ingredients or whole foods.

The safety evaluation of macronutrients or food components which comprise a substantial part of the diet, or of new processing technologies which have a potentially wide application, present special problems with regard to the design of feeding studies for toxicity testing. We have demonstrated that the application of a human-type diet with interchangeable macrocomponents is a feasible approach to address these issues.

Table 1
Composition of the Reference (AIN-76) and Human-type Diets

Component	AIN 76	Human-type
Industrial dry mix	–	88.9%
Casein	20.0%	–
Corn oil	10.0%	2.9%
Sugar	5.0%	5.0%
Cellulose	5.0%	–
Vitamin mix[1]	1.0%	1.0%
Mineral mix[2]	3.5%	2.0%
L-Methionine	0.3%	–
Choline bitartrate	0.2%	0.2%
Inositol	0.025%	0.025%
Corn starch	55.0%	–

[1] *Vitamin mixture (g or/IU/kg mix): thiamine-HCL (0.6 g), riboflavin (0.6 g), pyridoxine-HCL (0.7 g), nicotinic acid (3.0 g), Ca-D-pantothenate (1.6 g), folic acid (0.2 g), D-biotin (0.02 g), vitamin B12 (0.001 g), retinyl palmitate/acetate (400,000 IU), DL-alpha-tocopherol acetate (5000 IU), Vitamin D3 (100,000 IU), Vitamin K (0.005 g), and finely powdered sucrose to make to 1 kg.*

[2] *Mineral mixture (g/kg mix): calcium phosphate dibasic (500 g), sodium chloride (74 g), potassium citrate monohydrate (220 g), potassium sulphate (52 g), magnesium oxide (24 g), manganous carbonate (43-48% sulphate (52 g), magnesium oxide (24 g), manganous carbonate (43-48% Mn) (3.5 g), ferric citrate (16-17% Fe) (6 g), zinc carbonate (70% ZnO) (1.6 g), cupric carbonate (53-55%) Cu) (0.3 g), potassium iodate (0.01 g), sodium selenite (0.01 g), chromium potassium sulphate (0.55 g), and finely powdered sucrose to make to 1 kg.*

Table 2
Composition of the Industrial Dry Mix Used as a Base for the Human-type Diet

Product	%
Pre-cooked meat NC 27	23.63
Dehydrated mash potatoes	24.75
Lyophilized green beans	11.48
Carrots PD5mm	15.30
Lentils 5MTE 308131	7.77
Couscous	17.07

Table 3
Diet changes in haematological, clinical chemistry and organ weight values of rats fed the human-type diet (human) IN COMPARISON TO the reference AIN-76 diet (reference) for 13 weeks:

	Effect	Sex
Organ weights		
Liver weight	↑	M,(F)
Kidney weight	↑	M,F
Thymus weight	↓	F
Haematology		
Haemoglobin	↓	M,F
Mean platelet volume	↓	M,F
Blood biochemistry		
Bilirubin	↓	M,F
5'-Nucleotidase	↓	M,F
Amylase	↑	M
Potassium	↑	M
Iron	↓	M
Chloride	↑	M
Cholesterol	↓	M
Phospholipids	↓	M
Beta-globulins	↑	M
HDL	↓	M
LDL	↓	M

Table 4
Diet-related Histological Changes in Rats Fed the Human-type Diet in Comparison with AIN-76 (Reference Diet) after 13 Weeks

Tissue	Histological finding	Effect	Sex
Liver	cytoplasmic vacuolation of periportal hepatocytes hepatocellular "ground glass" cytoplasm	↓ ↑	M,F M
Kidney	cytoplasmic inclusions in single proximal tubules spontaneous corticomedullary mineralization	↑ ↓	M F
Urinary bladder	simple urothelial hyperplasia	↑	M,(F)
Spleen	haemosidrin-containing macrophages	↑	M,F

Figure 1
Comparison of the Macronutrient Composition of the Reference and Test (Human-type) Diets

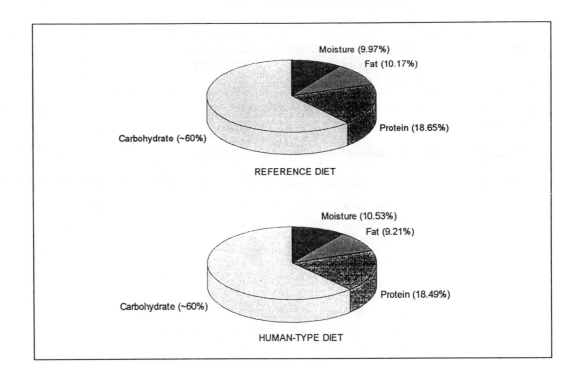

Figure 2
Evolution of body weight, food consumption and water consumption in male (circles) and female (squares) Sprague Dawley rats fed AIN-76 (control diet, open symbols) or the human-type diet (test diet, closed symbols). Values indicated are the mean of ten animals per group.

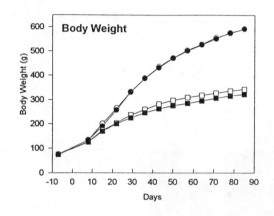
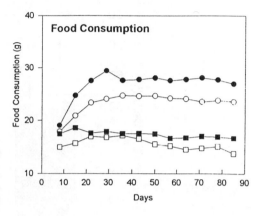
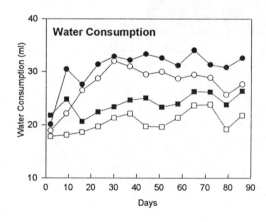

Figure 3
Effects of feeding the reference (striped bar) or human diet (hatched bar) on blood immunological values. Mean ±SD, n=20 (both sexes combined).

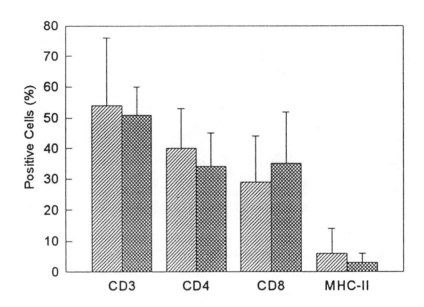

Figure 4

Effects of feeding the reference (striped bar) or human diet (hatched bar) on the activity of liver microsomal xenobiotic metabolizing enzymes and on the ability of the liver microsomal xenobiotic metabolizing enzymes and on the ability of the liver S9 fraction to activate (2-amino-3, 8-dimethylimidazo [4,5-*f*] quinoxaline) (MeIQx) to mutagenic metabolites in the Ames test. EROD: ethoxyresorufin O-deethylase; PROD: pentoxyresorufin O-deethylase; EMDM: erythromycin demethylase; ECOD: 7-ethoxycoumarin O-dethylase. Mean ±SD, n=10.

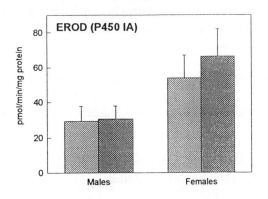
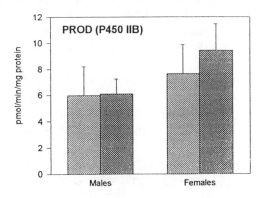
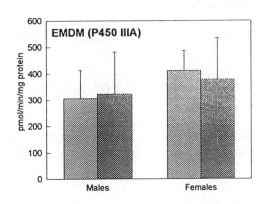
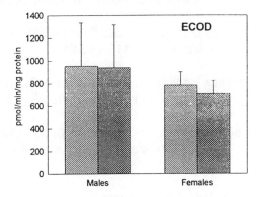
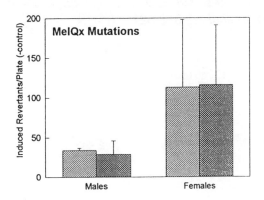

References

Alink, G.M., Kuiper, H.A., Beems, R.B. and Koeman, J.H. (1989) A study on the carcinogenicity of human diets in rats: The influence of heating and the addition of vegetables and fruit. *Fd. Chem. Toxic* 27:427-436.

American Institute of Nutrition (1977) Report of the American Institute of Nutrition ad hoc committee on standards for nutritional studies. *J. Nutr.* 107:1340-1348.

Burke, M.D., Thompson, S., Elcombe, C.R., Halpert, J., Haaparanta, T. and Mayer, R.T. (1985) Ethoxy-, pentoxy-, and benzyloxyphenoxazones and homologues: A series of substrates to distinguish between different induced cytochromes P-450. *Biochem. Pharmacol.* 34:3337-3345.

Greenlee, W.F., Poland, A. (1978) An improved assay of 7-ethoxycoumarin O-deethylase activity. Induction of hepatic enzyme activity in C57BL/6J and DBA/2J mice by phenobarbital, 3-methyl-cholanthrene and 2,3,7,8-tetrachlorodibenzo-p-dioxin. *J. Pharm. Exp. Ther.* 205:596-605.

Jonker, D. and Til, H.P. (1993) Sub-chronic (13-week) feeding study in rats with diets cooked by microwave or conventionally. TNO-report V 93.429.

Jones T.C., Mohr U. and Hunt R.D. (eds.) (1985) ILSI Monographs on Pathology of Laboratory Animals (Digestive System). Springer Verlag, New York.

Maron, D.M. and Ames, B.N. (1983) Revised methods for the salmonella mutagenicity test. *Mutat. Res.* 113:173-215.

Ritskes-Hoitinga J. and Beynen A.C. (1992) Nephrocalcinosis in the rat: A literature review. *Progress in Food and Nutrition Science* 16:85-124.

Tschantz, J.C. and Sunahara, G.I. (1993) Microaffinity chromatographic separation and characterization of lipoprotein fractions in rat and Mongolian gerbil serum. *Clin. Chem.* 39:1861-1867.

Wrighton, S.A., Schuetz, E.G., Watkins, P.B., Maurel, P., Barwick, J., Bailey, B.S., Hartle, H.T., Young, B. and Guzelian, P. (1985) Demonstration in multiple species of inducible hepatic cytochromes P-450 and their mRNAs related to the glucocorticoid-inducible cytochrome P-450 of the rat. *Mol. Pharmacol.* 28:312-321.

Investigations of the Allergenicity of Brazil Nut 2S Seed Storage Protein in Transgenic Soybean

**J.A. Nordlee, S.L. Taylor, J.A. Townsend,
L.A. Thomas and R. Townsend**

United States

Introduction

Seed storage proteins comprise an important part of the human and animal diet, but they are often deficient in certain essential amino acids. For example, seed storage proteins from legumes are typically deficient in sulfur containing amino acids. Soybean (*Glycine max*) meal that remains after oil extraction is a major animal feedstuff, but must be supplemented with synthetic methionine to ensure adequate animal nutrition. Similarly, human vegetarians must carefully balance their diets to avoid over-reliance on methionine-deficient legumes.

Many attempts have been made to improve the balance of essential amino acids in important crops through traditional methods of plant breeding (Bliss and Hall, 1977; Bright and Shewry, 1983). However, improvements in nutritional quality have often come at the expense of important agronomic properties such as yield or grain quality (Alexander, 1988). Methods based on recombinant DNA technology now afford opportunities to enhance the level of certain essential amino acids, without adversely affecting agronomic performance of a crop plant, by introducing genes into that crop from other plant species.

Seeds of the Brazil nut (*Bertholletia excelsa*) are unusually high in sulfur amino acids (about 8.3 per cent by weight). It has been recognized for many years that protein extracted from Brazil nut can serve as a methionine supplement for human food (Atunes and Markakes, 1977) and animal feed (Tao et al., 1987). Large scale use of Brazil nut for such purposes is clearly impracticable, but it is now possible to isolate a gene encoding a sulfur-rich protein from Brazil nut and transfer that gene to legume crops in order to improve their nutritional quality as either foods (Aragao et al., 1992; Saalbach et al., 1994) or feeds (Townsend et al., 1992).

A genomic clone encoding a 2S seed storage albumin protein, rich in methionine (18 per cent) and cysteine (8 per cent), was isolated from Brazil nut (Altenbach et al., 1987). The gene encodes a 17kD precursor polypeptide that is processed to 9kD and 3kD submits via a 12kD intermediate. In order to maximize expression of the 2S albumin in seeds of dicotyledonous plants, the 2S albumin precursor was placed under control of a seed specific promoter isolated from the phaseolin gene of *Phaseolus vulgaris*. The 2S seed storage albumin protein, rich in methionine (18 per cent) and cysteine (8 per cent), was isolated from Brazil nut (Altenbach et al., 1987). The gene encodes a 17kD precursor polypeptide that is processed to 9kD and 3kD subunits via a 12kD intermediate. In order to maximize expression of the 2S albumin in seeds of dicotyledonous plants, the 2S albumin precursor was placed under control of a seed specific promoter isolated from the phaseolin gene of *Phaseolus vulgaris*. The 2S albumin transgene was cloned into a disarmed *Agrobacterium* T-DNA vector carrying a selectable marker gene; neomycin phosphotransferase II (NPTII) and a visual marker gene; ß - glucuronidase (GUS), both under control of constitutive promoters. The vector was introduced into soybean using *Agrobacterium* mediated transformation (Townsend et al., 1992). Putative transformants were selected on kanamycin containing medium and recovered to the greenhouse where they were allowed to self-pollinate and set seed. Transformation was confirmed by Southern blot analysis of progeny using a DNA probe specific for the Brazil nut 2S albumin gene.

Seeds of transgenic soybean analyzed by SDS-PAGE contained high levels of a 9 kD protein that bound specifically to rabbit IgG raised against purified 2S albumin from Brazil nut. Transgenic plants were phenotypically and agronomically equivalent to untransformed controls and expression of the recombinant 2S albumin was stable in subsequent generations. Using a sensitive enzyme linked immunoassay for the 2S albumin, it was determined that the recombinant 2S albumin was stable in subsequent generations. Using a sensitive enzyme linked immunoassay for the 2S albumin, it was determined that the recombinant protein comprised approximately 4 to 8 per cent of the salt soluble protein fraction, equivalent to a 26 per cent gain in available methionine.

Brazil nut is recognized as a common cause of allergic reactions in a very small proportion of the population that is sensitive to tree-nuts (Gillespie et al., 1976; Arshad et al., 1991). The Food and Drug Administration (FDA) has identified allergenicity as a scientific issue relevant to public health and has directed developers of new plant varieties to consider the allergenic potential of the donor organism(s) in assessing the safety of foods derived from new plant varieties developed through methods such as recombinant DNA techniques (Anonymous, 1992). If there is insufficient information to demonstrate that an introduced protein could not cause an allergenic reaction in a susceptible population, then a label declaration is required to alert sensitive consumers.

Most soybeans are heat processed to extract oil. The protein fraction remains in the meal which is fed to animals. However, some soybean protein is also used in processed foods, for example as a protein "extender". It was important, therefore, to determine if recombinant Brazil nut 2S albumin expressed in transgenic soybean might be allergenic for Brazil nut sensitive individuals.

Materials and methods

Sera. Test sera were obtained from individuals with a documented history of allergic reactions to Brazil nut or avoidance of tree nuts. If these individuals consume Brazil nuts, they respond with symptoms that include swelling and itching in the oropharyngeal area, facial swelling, laryngeal edema and bronchospasm with wheezing. All individuals had positive skin prick tests to extracts of Brazil nut and their sera showed positive radioallergosorbant test (RAST), with binding to Brazil nut extracts of 9-64 times that of control sera from non-sensitive individuals. All individuals gave informed consent for these studies.

Seeds and proteins. Raw Brazil nuts were purchased from a local health store. Brazil nut 2S albumin was partially purified according to Sun et al., (1987). Transgenic soybean seed and seed of a genetically equivalent non-transgenic line were harvested from a small-scale, contained field trial conducted in 1993 in Polk, Iowa, in compliance with USDA-APHIS regulations. Purified NPTII and GUS were purchased commercially.

RAST inhibition. Fresh Brazil nut and soybean seeds were ground, defatted with acetone and di-ethyl ether and extracted into phosphate buffered saline and clarified by centrifugation. A Brazil nut solid phase was prepared (Aldolphson et al., 1986) using cyanogen bromide activated micro-crystalline cellulose and 10 mg of Brazil nut extract. Ten fold dilutions of Brazil nut and soybean extracts were reacted overnight with Brazil nut protein solid phase and pooled sera from four Brazil nut protein solid phase and pooled sera from four Brazil nut sensitive individuals. The solid phase was washed and then incubated with ^{125}Iodine labeled anti-human IgE. Excess labeled antibody was removed by washing and the radioactive counts bound to the solid phase were measured.

Immunoblotting. Partially purified Brazil nut 2S albumin and extracts from Brazil nut, transgenic soybean and non-transgenic soybean were separated by SDS-PAGE on 10-20 per cent gradient gels. The proteins were stained or electroblotted to nitrocellulose (Towbin et al., 1979). Blots were incubated with sera from nine Brazil nut sensitive individuals and bound IgE from the sera was detected with ^{125}Iodine labeled anti-human IgE and autoradiography.

Results

RAST inhibition. Proteins that bind IgE from allergic individuals are likely to be allergens. The extract from transgenic soybean was able to compete effectively with proteins extracted from raw Brazil nut bound to a solid phase, for binding to IgE from Brazil nut sensitive individuals. The inhibition was observed with comparable amounts of protein extracted from a genetically equivalent line of non-transformed soybean.

SDS-PAGE. Stained gels revealed the presence of a novel protein band in the transgenic soybean, corresponding to a molecular weight of approximately 9kD, which was also present in Brazil nut and comigrated with partially purified 2S albumin. An equivalent protein was absent from non-transformed soybean. Significant reductions in the staining intensity of certain proteins in the transgenic soybean were noted relative to the non-transgenic control.

Immunoblotting. Eight of the nine sera available in this study recognized the partially purified Brazil nut 2S albumin and also reacted with a protein of approximately 9 kD in the Brazil nut extract. Seven of the nine sera reacted with a 9kD protein in the transgenic soybean extract that comigrated with the Brazil nut 2S albumin. None of the sera reacted with any low molecular weight proteins in non-transgenic soybean, although sera from two individuals bound weakly to several higher molecular weight soybean proteins (i.e. in excess of 30 kD). There was no binding to purified NPTII or GUS. Sera from non-atopic control individuals did not react with any soybean or Brazil nut proteins.

Sera from four individuals bound weakly to several other Brazil nut proteins. Sera from two other individuals bound strongly to a 42 kD Brazil nut protein. One of these sera failed completely to react with 2S albumin or any protein in the transgenic soybean.

Five of the nine sera tested bound to a 12 kD protein that was present in some transgenic soybean extracts, but that was apparently absent from Brazil nut or the partially purified 2S albumin.

Discussion

The similarity between the RAST inhibition slopes of the two extracts from transgenic soybean and Brazil nut is indicative of a high degree of similarity between the IgE epitopes present in both seeds. Since inhibition is not due to cress reactions or non-specific binding to soybean protein (i.e. the non-transgenic soybean control produced no significant inhibition), we conclude that one or more allergens from Brazil nut have been introduced into the transgenic soybean.

Sera from eight of nine Brazil nut sensitive individuals bound strongly to purified Brazil nut 2S albumin and to a protein of similar molecular weight that was present in Brazil nut and soybean transformed with the Brazil nut 2S albumin gene, but absent from non-transformed soybean. We conclude that the 2S Brazil nut albumin is very likely a major allergen in Brazil nut and should be designated *Ber e*I (Marsh et al., 1987).

Confirmation of the allergenicity of *Ber e*I would require oral challenges with the 2S albumin. However, this could pose unacceptable risks to the group of patients who show life-threatening symptoms upon inadvertent consumption of Brazil nut. Since *Ber e*I retains its IgE binding capacity when expressed in transgenic soybean, it might elicit symptoms in Brazil nut sensitive individuals if they were to consume soybean protein containing the 2S albumin. Any food products derived from new plant varieties containing *Ber e*I should, therefore, be appropriately labeled to alert consumers, in accordance with FDA policy.

The existence of multiple IgE binding proteins in a single food is well known (Marsh et al., 1987). Peanut and soybean both contain multiple IgE binding proteins. In some instances these may reflect partially processed precursors of the mature allergen. In Brazil nut, the 2S albumin is known to be composed of 9 kD and 3 kD subunits that are processed from a 17 kD precursor protein via a 12 kD intermediate. In transgenic soybean, this processing often appears incomplete, resulting in the accumulation of the 12 kD intermediate (unpublished). The IgE binding epitope that is present on the 9 kD subunit is also conserved on the 12 kD intermediate, causing patient sera to recognize proteins. The 3 kD subunit either lacks an IgE binding epitope or was not retained on the gels. The existence of multiple epitopes would greatly complicate any attempts to eliminate the allergenicity of the 2S alumin by recombinant DNA manipulation.

This study demonstrates the value of RAST inhibition and SDS-PAGE with immunoblotting in the evaluation of the potential allergenicity of proteins produced by genes transferred from known allergenic material. However, we were only able to collect sera from nine individuals with allergies to Brazil nut although tree nuts are regarded as commonly allergenic foods. The availability of sera from patients with documented allergies to the source material places severe limitations on the application of these techniques to less common food allergens.

The majority of gene transfers in the field of plant biotechnology are from organisms that have no documented history of food use. These techniques will not be useful in predicting if these genes encode proteins that have the potential to be allergenic.

References

Adolphson, C.R., Gleich, G.J. and J.W. Yunginger (1986) In: N.R. Rose, H. Friedman and J.L. Fahey (eds.) *Manual of Clinical Laboratory Immunology*, pp. 652-659. American Society for Microbiology, Washington, D.C.

Alexander, D.E. (1988) Breeding special nutritional and industrial types. In: G.F. Sprague and J.W. Dudley (eds.) *Corn and Corn Improvement.* Agronomy Monograph No. 18, 3rd edition. American Society of Agronomy, Madison, Wisconsin, pp. 869-879.

Altenbach, S.B., Pearson, K.W., Marker, G., Staraci, L.C. and Sun, S.S.M. (1989) *Plant. Mol. Biol.* 13:513.

Anonymous (1992) Department of Health and Human Services – Food and Drug Administration statement of policy: Foods derived from new plant varieties. *Federal Register* 57:22984-23005.

Aragao, F.J.L., Grossi de Sa, M.F. and Almeida, E.R. (1992) *Plant Molecular Biology* 20:357-359.

Arshad, S.H., Malmberg, E., Kraft, K. and Hide, D.W. (1991) *Clinical and Experimental Allergy* 21:373.

Atunes, A.J. and Markakis, P. (1977) *J. Agric. Food Chem.* 25:1096.

Bliss, F.A. and Hall, T.C. (1977) *Cereal Food World* 22:106-113.

Bright, S.W.J. and Shewry, P.R. (1983) *CRC Critical Reviews in Plant Science* 1:49-93.

Gillespie, D.N., Nakajima, M.D.S. and Gleich, M.D. (1976) *J. Allergy Clin, Immunol.* 57:302.

Marsh, G.G., Goodfriend, L., King, T.P., Lowenstein, H. and Platts Mills, T.A.E. (1987) *J. Allergy Clin. Immunol.* 80:639.

Saalbach, I., et al. (1994) *Mol. Gen. Genet.* 242:226.

Sun, S.M., Leung, F.W. and Tomic, J.C. (1987) *Agric. Food, Chem.* 35:232.

Tao, S-H., et al. (1987) *Federation Proceedings* 46:891.

Towbin, H., Staelhelin, T. and Wallace, D.F.H. (1979) *Proc. Nat. Acad. Sci.* 76:4350.

Townsend, J.Á., et al. (1992) Proceeding of the 4th Biennial Conference on Molecular and Cellular Biology of Soybean, Iowa State University, Ames, Iowa, 27 July, p. 4.

US EPA Considerations for Mammalian Health Effects Presented by Transgenic Plant Pesticides[1]

John L. Kough

Biological Pesticides Section
Health Effects Division, Office of Pesticide Programs
United States Environmental Protection Agency

The Federal Insecticide, Fungicide and Rodenticide Act (FIFRA) gives the Environmental Protection Agency the responsibility for registering all pesticides prior to sale, distribution or use to prevent unreasonable adverse effects to humans and the environment. Under FIFRA a pesticide is defined as "...any substance or mixture of substances intended for preventing, destroying, repelling or mitigating any pest, or intended for use as a plant regulator, defoliant or desiccant..." The Office of Pesticide Programs (OPP) has responsibility for reviewing the safety of the product prior to FIFRA registration as a pesticide. In cooperation with the Food and Drug Administration, OPP also administers certain portions of the Federal Food Drug and Cosmetic Act (FFDCA) that relate to pesticide residues in food and feed.

OPP has as a working definition of a "plant pesticide" as a substance produced in a plant that is intended to act as a pesticide and the genetic material necessary to produce that pesticidal substance. It is important to note that OPP is not examining the plant *per se* but rather the pesticidal substance produced in the plant. The pesticidal substance itself (or pesticidal active ingredient) is the focus of the examination since it is the appropriate test substance for the mammalian safety evaluation. Within OPP, the Health Effects Division reviews areas of the safety evaluation of plant pesticides related to mammalian toxicology and the Environmental Fate and Effects Division reviews areas related to the environmental fate of the plant pesticide and its non-target toxicology.

For product assessment, OPP has divided the pesticidal active ingredients into two categories: proteinaceous and non-proteinaceous pesticides. This approach is based on the fact that plant proteins, whether characterized or not, are a significant component of the human diet and are susceptible to acid and enzymatic digestion prior to assimilation. Presuming the new proteinaceous products are adequately characterized, minimum human health concerns would exist unless 1) the proteins have been implicated in mammalian toxicity; 2) human exposure to the protein, although never implicated in mammalian toxicity through different routes of exposure, has not been documented; or 3) "novel" proteins are created via modification of the primary structure of the natural protein pesticide. Non-

---

[1] This paper summarizes a paper by J.T. McClintock, R.D. Sjoblad and R. Engler entitled "Toxicological Evaluation of Genetically Engineered Plant Pesticides", Chapter 5 in *Food Safety Assessment*, American Chemical Society Symposium Series No. 484, 1992.

proteinaceous plant pesticides may be evaluated separately, perhaps in a manner analogous to that for conventional chemical or biochemical pesticides.

The main intent of this talk is to discuss the fundamental information needed to assess the human health risks associated with the widespread use and distribution of transgenic plants modified to produce new pesticidal products. Fundamental to this evaluation is a thorough description of the source and nature of the pesticidal substance, including the source of the inserted genes or gene sequences necessary to produce the pesticide and any novel proteins encoded by this genetic material. Presuming that these proteins have been adequately characterized, this information would allow a reasonable prediction of the toxicology issues and the type of data necessary to evaluate the potential risks. The Health Effects Division evaluates two areas of information relating to the plant pesticide: product characterization and mammalian toxicology.

Product characterization

Characterization of the plant pesticide covers four areas: 1) identification of the donor organism(s) and the gene sequence(s) inserted into the recipient plant; 2) identification and description of the vector or delivery system used to move the gene into the recipient plant; 3) identification of the recipient organism, including information on the insertion of the gene sequence; and 4) data and information on the level of expression of the pesticidal substance. This information is critical for assessing potential risks resulting from exposure of humans and domestic animals to the plant pesticide.

Source of genetic material encoding the plant pesticide

1) Identity of the donor organism(s) using current taxonomy and the most sensitive and specific methods available.

2) Identity of the genetic material encoding the pesticidal substance (or proteins involved in producing the pesticidal substance if a non-proteinaceous pesticide).

Pesticidal substances

1) Identity and characterization of the proteins/peptides encoded by the inserted genetic material.

2) Identity and characterization of the non-proteinaceous pesticidal substance resulting from the inserted sequences.

Vector system

1) A description of the vectors, the identity of the organisms used for cloning of the vectors, and a description of the methodologies used to construct all the vectors. This vector description should include the size in kilobases, appropriate restriction endonuclease sites, location and function of all relevant gene segments, all

modifications (e.g. deletions of transposition functions, restriction site alterations and disarming the Ti plasmid), and the final delivery system itself.

2) A description of the gene segment(s) actually transferred to the plant.

Recipient plant

1) Identity and taxonomy of the recipient plant including cultivars and lines if applicable.

2) A description of significant characteristics including i) any previous modifications, ii) life cycle, iii) mode of reproduction and dissemination, and iv) geographical distribution and wild relatives.

3) A description of the methods used to deliver the gene sequence to the plant and confirm its stable insertion.

Gene expression in the plant

1) A description of whether the inserted genes are expressed constitutively or inducibly; localization and expression of the pesticidal substance in plant parts; and an estimation of the gene copies inserted.

2) Gene expression during the life cycle.

Product analysis and residue chemistry

1) The proposed mode of action of the pesticidal substance

2) Concentrations of the pesticidal substance in the plant and plant parts and the analytical methods used to quantify these.

Physical and chemical properties

For plant producing non-proteinaceous pesticidal substances, data or information relating to the chemical or physical properties may be relevant for the risk assessment.

Toxicology

The information cited above can be used to establish what the necessary mammalian toxicology data would be to determine potential risks associated with human and domestic exposure to transgenic plant pesticidal substances. Some of the key factors would be if the pesticide was proteinaceous or not, and whether the use pattern will result in dietary and/or non-dietary exposure. To illustrate these points, certain categories of plant pesticides have been created here and their potential risk endpoints described. The first category (I) includes plants engineered to produce proteinaceous pesticides that have never been produced by plants such as the δ-endotoxin from *Bacillus thuringiensis*. The second category (II) could include plants engineered to produce pesticidal substances from other plants which may or may not be proteinaceous. Examples of this category would include proteins involved in producing secondary metabolites found in other plants, digestive enzyme inhibitors, and perhaps a synthetic gene producing a pesticidal substance. The third category (III) would be plants engineered to produce *de novo* a non-proteinaceous pesticidal substance.

The dietary consumption is presumed to be the predominant route of exposure for food and feed crops engineered to express pesticidal substances. For all food or feed crops producing proteinaceous pesticidal substances (i.e. categories I and/or II), mammalian toxicology could be assessed by acute oral studies (**Table 1**). The assessment of dermal irritation/toxicity might be addressed through reporting of any adverse reactions from skin contact during product development or use. Reporting of dermal effects resulting from incidental exposure may also suffice for non-food uses, depending on the extent of skin exposure.

For plants genetically engineered to produce a non-proteinaceous pesticide (i.e. categories II and/or III) and intended for food or feed use, the primary route of exposure would again be dietary (Table 1). The potential toxicity of the pesticidal substances could also be assessed by oral toxicity studies (acute, subchronic or chronic feeding studies). If plants in categories II and III were engineered to produce volatile pesticide components, pulmonary exposure might be significant even without a food use. Dermal exposure to non-proteinaceous pesticides products in categories II and III may also be limited to the reporting of dermal effects, depending on extent of exposure.

The limited routes of significant exposure to transgenic plant pesticides should simplify the appropriate toxicology testing necessary for pesticide registration. As outlined above, it is evident that proteinaceous pesticides would have a reduced set of toxicology endpoints to address compared to non-proteinaceous pesticides. This is again based on the anticipated degradation of these proteinaceous compounds to amino acids with passage through the gastrointestinal tract. The fundamental framework for assessing the potential toxicological issues with plant pesticides depends to a large extent on the product characterization data and related information. **Table 2** provides a summary of the information that would be relevant for these purposes.

Other issues and concerns

As "plant pesticides" have been defined for FIFRA, products that are intentionally added along with the pesticidal genes are considered inert ingredients. These inert ingredients, generally termed marker genes, are used early in the plant cell transformation process to identify those cells successfully incorporating the desired plant pesticidal gene. Many of the same considerations discussed above would also relate to the proteins or other substances expressed as inert ingredients (i.e. marker genes).

OPP has also suggested that it may be appropriate to develop an *in vitro* digestibility assay to assess the potential of proteins to be degraded in the presence of gastric or intestinal fluids. The assumption on which this test is based is that proteins that are rapidly degraded in a simulated gastrointestinal exposure would also be unlikely to express toxicity by the oral route. This test could have wider applicability for screening modified proteins once a correlation between the results of the *in vitro* digestibility assay and the acute oral toxicity test were established.

Table 1
Potential Mammalian Toxicology Requirements

Plant category	Intended use	Data requirements
Category I and II (peroteinaceous pesticidal substances only)		
	Food	Acute oral; reporting of observed dermal effects
	Non-food	Reporting of observed dermal effects
Category II and III (non-proteinaceous pesticidal substances)		
	Food	Oral studies (acute, subchronic or chronic feeding studies); reporting of observed dermal effects; pulmonary studies[a]
	Non-food	Reporting of observed dermal effects; pulmonary studies

[a] *Only if the plant pesticidal substance has significant inhalation exposure or is volatile*

Table 2
Summary of Data and Information Necessary for the Evaluation of Transgenic Plants Expressing Pesticidal Properties

Discipline	Proteinaceous		Non-proteinaceous	
	Food	Non-food[a]	Food	Non-food[a]
Product characterization	X	X	X	X
Expected human exposure				
Oral	X	O	X	O
Pulmonary	O	O	X[b]	X[b]
Dermal[c]	O	O	O	O

X = Data and/or information necessary

O = Data and/or information not needed

[a] Members of this category may include certain engineered plants whose pesticidal substances and intentionally added inserts have been shown not to have significant human exposure

[b] Only if the pesticidal substance has been shown to have significant pulmonary exposure or is volatile

[c] Reporting of adverse effects resulting from dermal exposure may be sufficient

ANNEX I

REPORT OF THE WORKING GROUP SESSIONS

Introduction

This Workshop was convened by the OECD to address the safety of new foods from plant, animal and microbial origins. To facilitate discussion of the papers presented in the preceding part of this report, two Working Groups were established. The discussions in the two Working Groups developed in a supplementary way, and therefore their reports are combined in this section of the report. The combined report has been agreed by the Chairmen of the Working Groups as a fair compilation of the points raised and discussed, but should not be regarded as a consensus view of all participants.

A number of aspects relating to the safety evaluation of new foods were considered, including: application of the principle of substantial equivalence; the various analytical *in vitro* and *in vivo* studies that might be used in food safety assessment; and issues associated with novel microorganisms used in food production.

A. Use of substantial equivalence in food safety assessment

Three situations were considered:

1) There is substantial equivalence between the new food and a traditional counterpart (e.g. virus-resistant plants produced by insertion of the viral coat protein, or herbicide-tolerant plants produced by introducing a protein comparable to one already present in the plant but tolerant to a selective herbicide);

2) There is substantial equivalence between the new food and a traditional counterpart, except for the inserted trait (e.g. insect-protected plants produced by introduction of a *Bt* gene or disease-resistant plants produced by introduction of a new protein); and

3) Substantial equivalence between the new food and a traditional counterpart does not exist (e.g. introduction of a gene or genes that encode a trait that significantly alters the plant for use in food or feed, such as production of a new oil or carbohydrate).

It was concluded that the same approach could be applied in establishing substantial equivalence in respect to foods and food components from plants, animals and microorganisms.

Substantial equivalence

The concept of "substantial equivalence", as elaborated by the OECD, embodies the idea that existing organisms used as food, or as a source of food, can be used as the basis for comparison when assessing the safety for human consumption of a food or food component that has been modified or is new. Several interpretations of the term "substantial equivalence" were noted. It was agreed that an appropriate strategy for the determination of substantial equivalence could be developed only with a clear understanding of the way in which the term was being interpreted. Substantial equivalence is related to the composition of the ingested product in terms of nutritional, antinutritional and functional characteristics in comparison to the traditional counterpart. Substantial equivalence must be a dynamic concept, since the basis of comparison (e.g. the traditional counterpart) will expand as new products, including genetically modified plant products, are introduced.

The purpose of determining substantial equivalence is two-fold: to allow an assumption of safety comparative to the traditional counterpart; and to identify what aspects of the product, if any, require further study. Substantial equivalence may be applied narrowly to show that, apart from the intended modification, there are no untoward effects by comparison to the parent organism. In the broader application, comparison to the parent may not be sufficient; substantial equivalence would be developed by considering the range, for a given compound or component, for commercial food varieties of the species under consideration.

The establishment of substantial equivalence also leads to a conclusion of equivalent wholesomeness in comparison to the parent as well as to the species in the broader sense. Wholesomeness in this context covers protection of human health and well-being.

Key components for a given product are the focus in determining substantial equivalence. Data bases provide a useful tool in establishing substantial equivalence through characterization of type and range of content of chemical constituents such as natural toxicants, nutrients and antinutritional factors. Phenotypic and agronomic characteristics are also components in establishing substantial equivalence.

Once substantial equivalence is established, the product should be considered as safe as its traditional counterpart.

Substantial equivalence except for the inserted trait

When the product is substantially equivalent to a traditional counterpart except for the inserted trait, it was concluded that further safety assessment should focus on the product of the inserted gene. The toxicity of the DNA and mRNA *per se* is not an issue. However, the stability of the gene insert/construct and the potential for transfer (particularly for microorganisms) are relevant issues in the assessment.

The approach to evaluation should be case-by-case and based on established knowledge and the characterization of the introduced gene(s) and gene product(s) including (list is not exhaustive):

- source
- identity
- construction
- effect
- digestibility (degree of digestibility)
- stability of the trait

- protein and any products of its action (secondary metabolites)
- site of expression (tissue specificity)
- colonization potential (microorganisms)

These aspects were not discussed in detail apart from digestibility. When the protein(s) expressed by the introduced gene(s) is/are shown to be rapidly digested and is/are not derived from a source(s) known to be allergenic (see section E, Allergenicity), no further analysis of the safety of the expressed protein should be required. However, in situations where a protein is poorly digested, its intended cellular function will need to be assessed from a safety point of view. Furthermore, poor digestibility may be an indicator of potential toxicity or allergenicity which needs to be addressed in further studies. These may entail *in vitro* testing and/or metabolic studies including absorption and distribution. The need for further testing should be determined by applying a sequential approach. A decision tree would be useful in determining how a product might move to more testing. Even when a protein is shown to be poorly digested, it may not be necessary for protein products to undergo animal testing. However, when pursuing animal testing, the objectives must be clear and experiments designed with care.

Not substantially equivalent

Food items considered not to be substantially equivalent might include: novel food plants, animals or microorganisms; new single cell proteins; new macro-nutrients such as fat replacers and sugar substitutes. Just because a new food is not substantially equivalent to an existing food does not mean that it is less safe, but that safety testing that would be required should be based on the properties of the new food. On the basis of the chemical composition and familiarity, some assumptions can be made regarding the necessity of animal studies and *in vitro* studies (in particular, genotoxicity).

A sequential approach should be used to determine the appropriate testing strategy for such a new product. Not all products may require animal testing and should therefore be assessed on a case-by-case basis. If animal studies with food or food components are deemed appropriate, their objectives must be clear and care taken in experimental design.

B. Analytical Studies

The history of safe use of a food or food component provides the baseline for determining substantial equivalence. The assessment of intended and unintended effects as the result of, for example, any genetic modification should be directed by existing knowledge of the organism. For intended changes, primary consideration should be focused on the nature of the transferred genetic material and on any new gene products produced (e.g. protein). In addition, targeted alterations of well-characterized metabolic pathways (e.g. herbicide tolerance) or of food composition (e.g. modified vegetable oil) should be used to focus the evaluation on changes in plant biochemistry.

Assessment of unintended changes, that is, changes that are not predicted based on the introduced gene(s) or gene product(s), will require a thorough knowledge of the biology of the system in determining the need for analytical studies. While the inserted genetic material is well-characterized, generally the site of insertion or potential effects of the insertion event on the plant genome cannot be readily assessed. However, unintended effects may occur as a result of all methods of plant breeding. Plant breeders already have screening systems to eliminate "offtypes" that do not conform to standard or accepted specifications of the marketplace. For instance, data on composition commonly generated for new plant varieties for variety registration could serve as the basis of this comparative analyses. Evaluation of genetically modified plant varieties should also include the consideration of agronomic characteristics, which may reflect unintended effects. This provides some assurance of the lack of significant pleiotropic effects. In most cases, it may be desirable to provide assurance that unintended, undesirable changes have not occurred in the concentration of key nutrients, toxicants and anti-nutrients in the finished food.

Complicating factors for these analyses may include a lack of information on composition and on natural variation of important nutrients and toxicants for comparative purposes. Along with the absence of historical data, the lack of standardized analytical methodology and its expense were also noted, particularly in the case of minor crops.

C. Data bases

Data bases can provide valuable baseline information on the composition of foods. They can provide valuable reference points for assessing whether significant changes have occurred in key nutrients and toxicants. Consideration should also be given to the ranges of significant toxicants and nutrients in commercially acceptable plant varieties. Furthermore, the quality of data must be assured and validated methods should be developed for quantifying key components. However, these data bases should not become checklists of the parameters that should be measured, since evidence is accumulating that some of the compounds previously considered to be toxicants may actually play nutritional or anti-cancer roles.

D. *In vitro* and *in vivo* testing

Toxicological tests may be indicated in cases where safety questions cannot be resolved using genetic, molecular, chemical and agronomic data and information. In those cases where toxicological studies are needed in order to complete the safety assessment, *in vitro* and *in vivo* bioassays may be used. *In vitro* studies are particularly useful with respect to elucidation of mechanisms of toxic action of compounds. While it may be desirable to use *in vitro* assays, proper validation of such systems is essential to avoid confounding results.

The initial assessment of proteins *per se*, expressed as a result of genetic modification, should focus on *in vitro* digestibility. Proteins that are digestible and have no record of toxicity in higher vertebrates are unlikely to require further toxicological testing. In general, proteins introduced by genetic modification will not pose problems for special groups (immuno-compromised, infants and geriatrics) because they are microconstituents of the food.

In cases where the safety of proteins introduced by genetic modification cannot be established by assessment of the digestibility, function or toxicity of the protein, carefully designed toxicological studies on the protein may be needed. One industry representative noted that, based on his experience to date, the preferred test material is the protein produced in an appropriate fermentation system that generates a protein substantially equivalent to the protein that is found in the plant.

Testing of whole foods in animals is not generally recommended for foods derived as a result of genetic modification of food crops and will, in general, be required only for those which cannot be shown to be substantially equivalent to their traditional counterparts. It was recognized that there are difficulties in the testing of whole foods. Animal feeding studies in general are not sensitive enough to detect unintended effects as a result of gene modification. Therefore, if animal studies are considered necessary, there is a need to modify existing protocols for testing food or food components, in particular by providing adequate nutrition with respect to diet. The usual concept of safety margins may not be applicable.

The concept of the wholesomeness of the food needs to be applied. The wholesomeness concept demands well-designed animal studies where concern related to nutritional imbalance is addressed. Nutritional imbalance may mask toxic effects (e.g. increase in exposure may result in imbalance; if the diet is marginal, addition of test material might shift diet into imbalance, i.e. deficiency or excess).

Consideration could be given to the testing of extracts rather than whole food. The results from such studies may give clues as to what might constitute a toxicological concern. Testing of extracts in isolation may be problematic in that interpretation may be complicated in predicting effects for the whole food. The absence of a traditional counterpart for a novel food complicates the interpretation, though a dose-response analysis might prove effective in counteracting this (i.e. might provide a safety factor). The testing of specific components of a novel food may also present an option for addressing safety testing.

Human evaluation of organoleptic properties of foods is a routine procedure in the development of vegetable crops. However, these studies, which are often limited to "sip and spit" tests, are typically considered part of the product quality assessment, not the safety assessment of these products. Therefore, once the initial safety assessment has been completed for a food product, sensory evaluations should be conducted as these evaluations would typically be performed for the quality and consumer acceptance evaluation for that product.

Human studies may be appropriate for safety assessment in those specific cases where there is reason to believe that particular groups in the population, e.g. immuno-compromised individuals, infants and geriatrics, may metabolize the novel food in ways that are not typical of the general population or may consume excessive quantities of a particular foodstuff.

E. Allergenicity

It is known that a very small number of foods contain major allergens. Tests exist to identify the gene products responsible for causing these adverse reactions in the small proportion of the population affected. In considering the safety of novel foods, attention should therefore be given to the origin of the inserted gene.

If the gene is obtained from a food organism which is not known to be allergenic, the probability of the introduced protein being allergenic is remote. There are, at present, no predictive tests for assessing potential allergenicity of proteins from sources that are not commonly recognized as allergens. While it is unlikely that a protein will elicit an allergic reaction, a comparison of the properties of the introduced protein with those of known allergens may prove valuable in minimizing the likelihood that the new protein will be an allergen. Among the criteria which should be considered are: molecular weight in the region of 10 to 70 kD, similarity of amino acid sequence to known allergens, resistance to digestion and heat denaturation, glycosylation, and relative abundance. Human experiences in terms of allergenicity are also relevant.

In general, it was concluded that the assumption can be made that a protein is not likely to be allergenic unless its properties suggest the possibility.

F. Exotic foods

Attention should be paid to new exotic foods introduced onto new markets. In these cases, history of safe use of such products in another country should be taken into account.

G. Special issues for microorganisms

The expertise in the Working Groups lay primarily in the area of food plants. In relation to foods obtained from microorganisms, it was felt that much of the foregoing discussion also applied. However, for products of microbial origin, there were further factors that might need to be taken into account. The safety consideration should be based on the way in which the microorganism would be used, its biology, and its history of use in food processing. Where the organism has an extensive history of use in food processing, the primary consideration for safety assessment would focus on ensuring that the final product does not contain unacceptable contaminants. It is important to consider if the microorganism has a history of safe use for food production irrespective of whether or not it occurs in the final food. It might be useful to consider the development of a list of microorganisms acceptable for use in food or in the production of food. In view of the potential for new microorganisms consumed as food to colonize the gut or to transfer genes to the gut microflora, it was considered that attention should be given to the development and validation of models to assess these aspects in relation to genetically modified microorganisms.

ANNEX II

LIST OF PARTICIPANTS

OECD Workshop on Food Safety Evaluation
Oxford, England
12-15 September 1994

Austria

Mr Edmund Plattner
Toxicology/Bio-technology Division
Federal Ministry of Health, Sports and Consumer Protection

Belgium

Dr N. Delzenne
Université Catholique de Louvain
Unité BCTC

Canada

Dr Paul R. Mayers
Head, Office of Food Biotechnology
Evaluation Division, Bureau of Microbial Hazards
Food Directorate
Health Protection Branch

Czech Republic

Ing Helena Stepánková
Institute of Biotechnology

Denmark

Dr Bodil Lund Jacobsen
National Food Agency of Denmark
Institute of Toxicology

Dr Ib Knudsen
Head of Institute DVM
National Food Agency of Denmark

Finland

Dr Anja Hallikainen
National Food Administration

France

Dr Christina Collet-Ribbing
CNERNA-CNRS

Germany

Prof Dr Walter P. Hammes
Hohenheim University
Institute of Food Technology

Dr Joachim Bollmann
Federal Ministry of Agriculture,
Food and Forestry

Dr F. Laplace
Federal Ministry of Science and Technology

Dr Marianna Schauzu
Federal Institute for Health Related
Consumer Protection and Veterinary Medicine

Dr Ralf Greiner
Federal Research Centre for Nutrition

Greece

Dr Spyridon B. Litsas
General Secretariat of Research and Technology

Italy

Dr Marina Miraglia
Istituto Superiore de Sanita

Japan

Dr Akihiro Hino
Department of Biotechology
Ministry of Agriculture, Forestry and Fisheries

Dr Seizo Sumida
Director, Safety and Environment
Japan Bioindusty Association

Mr Shoji Tsubuku
Life Science Laboratories
Central Research Laboratories
Ajinomoto Co, Inc.

Mr Ken-Ichi Hayashi
Society for Techno-Innovation of Agriculture, Forestry and Fisheries

Dr Masatake Toyoda
National Institute of Hygienic Sciences

Mexico

Dr Amanda Galvez-Mariscal
Facultad de Quimica
Universidad Nacional Autonoma de Mexico

Netherlands

Mr Harry Kuiper
State Institute for Quality Control of Agricultural Products (RIKILT-DLO)

Dr Esther J. Kok
State Institute for Quality Control of Agricultural Products (RIKILT-DLO)

Dr Frans van Dam
Consumer and Biotechnology Foundation

Dr P.M. Andreoli
Gist-Brocades

Norway

Ms Svanhild Foldal
Norwegian Biotechnology Advisory Board

Professor Tore Aune
Norwegian College of Veterinary Medicine

Spain

Dr Antonio de Castro
Instituto de la Grasa - CSIC

Dr Daniel Ramon-Vidal
Instituto Agroquamica y Tecnologia de Alimentos

Switzerland

Dr Karoline Dorsch-Hesler
Swiss Committee for Biosafety

Dr Josef Schlatter
Federal Office of Public Health
Food Science Division
C/o Institute of Toxicology

Dr Anthony C. Huggett
Nestec Ltd.

United Kingdom

Ms Ranjini Rasaiah
Ministry of Agriculture, Fisheries and Food

Dr David Jonas
Ministry of Agriculture, Fisheries and Food

Ms Sue O'Hagan
Department of Health

Mrs Carol James
British Society of Plant Breeders Ltd

Mrs Sue Hattersley
Department of Health

Miss Pendi Najran
Ministry of Agriculture, Fisheries and Food

Dr Norman Lazarus
Department of Health

Dr Peter J. Rodgers
Zeneca Bio Products

Dr Maurice Smith
Unilever Environmental Safety Laboratory

Dr Michael Nelson
Kings College (KQC)
University of London

United States

Dr Bruce Hammond
Monsanto Company, C2SE

Dr Roy Fuchs
Monsanto Company, GG4J

Dr James H. Maryanski
Strategic Manager for Biotechnology
Center for Food Safety and Applied Nutrition
FDA

Dr Rod Townsend
Pioneer Hi-Bred Int. Inc.

Ms Sharynne George Nenon
The United States Mission to the EU

Dr David G. Hattan
Division of Health Effects Evaluation HFS-225
Center for Food Safety and Applied Nutrition
FDA

Dr John L. Kough
US EPA Office of Pesticide Programs

Dr Hector Quemada
Asgrow Seed Company/Upjohn

European Commission

Dr K. Mehta
European Commission

Dr K. Schreiber
European Commission

OECD Secretariat

Dr Peter Kearns
Environmental Health and Safety Division

Dr Herman B.W.M. Koëter
Environmental Health and Safety Division

Ms Lisa Zannoni
Environmental Health and Safety Division

Dr Mark Cantley
Directorate for Science, Technology and Industry

Dr Yoshitika Ando
Directorate for Science, Technology and Industry

Mr Yoshinobu Miyamura
Directorate for Science, Technology and Industry

Dr Muriel Dunier
Directorate for Food, Agriculture and Fisheries

OECD Environmental Health and Safety Publications

<u>List as of April 1996</u>

**OECD Environment Directorate,
Environmental Health and Safety Division**

**2 rue André-Pascal
75775 Paris Cedex 16
FRANCE**

Fax: (33-1) 45 24 16 75

E-mail: ehscont@oecd.org

For more information, and the full text of some of these publications, consult the OECD's World Wide Web site (http://www.oecd.org/ehs/)

Please note:

[F] *following a title indicates the entire publication is <u>available from the OECD in a separate French translation</u>. The other publications listed are available in English only, but they normally include a French summary.*

[GLP] *following a title indicates the publication is part of the OECD Series on Principles of Good Laboratory Practice and Compliance Monitoring. Translations of this series into German, Russian, Polish, Czech, Slovak, Hebrew, Spanish and Italian exist or are planned. For more information, please contact the Environmental Health and Safety Division.*

The OECD Environment Monograph series:

The Environment Monograph series makes technical documents prepared by the OECD Environment Directorate available to the public. The Environment Monographs on this list were prepared by the Environmental Health and Safety Division. Copies are available upon request at no charge, in limited quantities.

No. 14, *Final Report of the Expert Group on Model Forms of Agreement for the Exchange of Confidential Data on Chemicals* (1988)[F]

No. 15, *Final Report of the Working Group on Mutual Recognition of Compliance with Good Laboratory Practice* (1988)[F]

No. 17, *The Use of Industry Category Documents in Source Assessment of Chemicals* (1989)[F]

No. 24, *Accidents Involving Hazardous Substances* (1989)[F]

No. 26, *Report of the OECD Workshop on Ecological Effects Assessment* (1989)[F]

No. 27, *Compendium of Environmental Exposure Assessment Methods for Chemicals* (1989)[F]

No. 28, *Workshop on Prevention of Accidents Involving Hazardous Substances: Good Management Practice* (1990)[F]

No. 29, *Workshop on the Provision of Information to the Public and on the Role of Workers in Accident Prevention and Response* (1990)[F]

No. 30, *Workshop on the Role of Public Authorities in Preventing Major Accidents and in Major Accident Land-Use Planning* (1990)[F]

No. 31, *Workshop on Emergency Preparedness and Response and on Research in Accident Prevention, Preparedness and Response* (1990)[F]

No. 35, *A Survey of New Chemicals Notification Procedures in OECD Member Countries* (1990)[F]

No. 36, *Scientific Criteria for Validation of In Vitro Toxicity Tests* (1990)[F]

No. 39, *International Survey on Biotechnology Use and Regulations* (1990)[F]

[no number] *Users Guide to Hazardous Substance Data Banks Available in OECD Member Countries*, OCDE/GD(91)102 (1991)[F]

[Also translated into Spanish by the United Nations Environment Programme's Industry and Environment Office (UNEP IE).]

[no number] *Users Guide to Information Systems Useful to Emergency Planners and Responders Available in OECD Member Countries*, OCDE/GD(91)103 (1991)[F]

[Also translated into Spanish by UNEP IE.]

No. 43, *International Directory of Emergency Response Centres* (1992)[F]

[The International Directory is a co-operative project of OECD and UNEP IE. The emergency response centres listed in this Directory are located in both OECD and non-OECD countries.]

No. 44, *Workshop on Prevention of Accidents Involving Hazardous Substances: The Role of the Human Factor in Plant Operations* (1992)

No. 45, *The OECD Principles of Good Laboratory Practice* (1992)[F, GLP]

No. 46, *Guides for Compliance Monitoring Procedures for Good Laboratory Practice* (1992)[F, GLP]

[superseded by No. 110, *Revised Guides for Compliance Monitoring Procedures for Good Laboratory Practice* (1995)]

No. 47, *Guidance for the Conduct of Laboratory Inspections and Study Audits* (1992)[F, GLP]

[superseded by No. 111, *Revised Guidance for the Conduct of Laboratory Inspections and Study Audits* (1995)]

No. 48, *Quality Assurance and GLP* (1992)[F, GLP]

No. 49, *Compliance of Laboratory Suppliers with GLP Principles* (1992)[F, GLP]

No. 50, *The Application of the GLP Principles to Field Studies* (1992)[F, GLP]

No. 51, *Guiding Principles for Chemical Accident Prevention, Preparedness and Response: Guidance for Public Authorities, Industry, Labour and Others for the Establishment of Programmes and Policies related to Prevention of, Preparedness for, and Response to Accidents Involving Hazardous Substances* (1992)[F]

[The Guiding Principles are also available in Russian. They are being translated into Spanish, and may also be translated into other languages. For more information, please contact the Environmental Health and Safety Division.]

No. 52, *Report of the OECD Workshop on Monitoring of Organisms Introduced into the Environment* (1992)

No. 58, *Report of the OECD Workshop on Quantitative Structure Activity Relationships (QSARS) in Aquatic Effects Assessment* (1992)

No. 59, *Report of the OECD Workshop on the Extrapolation of Laboratory Aquatic Toxicity Data to the Real Environment* (1992)

No. 60, *Report of the OECD Workshop on Effects Assessment of Chemicals in Sediment* (1992)

No. 65, *Risk Reduction Monograph No. 1: Lead* (1993)

No. 66, *Report of the OECD Workshop on Strategies for Transporting Dangerous Goods by Road: Safety and Environmental Protection* (1993)

[The OECD's Chemical Accidents Programme and Road Transport Research Programme co-operated in organising this workshop.]

No. 67, *Application of Structure-Activity Relationships to the Estimation of Properties Important in Exposure Assessment* (1993)

No. 68, *Structure-Activity Relationships for Biodegradation* (1993)

No. 69, *Report of the OECD Workshop on the Application of Simple Models for Exposure Assessment* (1993)

No. 70, *Occupational and Consumer Exposure Assessments* (1993)

No. 73, *The Application of the GLP Principles to Short-term Studies* (1993)[F, GLP]

No. 74, *The Role and Responsibilities of the Study Director in GLP Studies* (1993)[F, GLP]

No. 76, *OECD Series on the Test Guidelines Programme No. 1: Guidance Document for the Development of OECD Guidelines for Testing of Chemicals* (1993; reformatted 1995)[F]

No. 77, *Data Requirements for Pesticide Registration in OECD Member Countries: Survey Results* (1993)

No. 81, *Health Aspects of Chemical Accidents: Guidance on Chemical Accident Awareness, Preparedness and Response for Health Professionals and Emergency Responders* (1994)[F]

[Four international organisations collaborated in the preparation of this publication: the International Programme on Chemical Safety (IPCS), OECD, UNEP IE, and the World Health Organization – European Centre for Environment and Health (WHO-ECEH).]

No. 88, *US EPA/EC Joint Project on the Evaluation of (Quantitative) Structure Activity Relationships* (1994)

No. 90: *Ottawa '92: The OECD Workshop on Methods for Monitoring Organisms in the Environment* (1994)*

No. 91: *Compendium of Methods for Monitoring Organisms in the Environment* (1994)*

[*Monographs No. 90 and 91 are companion documents.]

No. 92, *Guidance Document for Aquatic Effects Assessment* (1995)

No. 93, *Report of the OECD Workshop on Chemical Safety in Port Areas* (1994)

[This Workshop was co-sponsored by OECD, the International Maritime Organization (IMO) and UNEP.]

No. 94, *Report of the OECD Special Session on Chemical Accident Prevention, Preparedness and Response at Transport Interfaces* (1995)

No. 95, *Report of the OECD Workshop on Small and Medium-sized Enterprises in Relation to Chemical Accident Prevention, Preparedness and Response* (1995)

No. 98, *OECD Series on the Test Guidelines Programme No. 2: Detailed Review Paper on Biodegradability Testing* (1995)

No. 99, *Commercialisation of Agricultural Products Derived through Modern Biotechnology: Survey Results* (1995)

No. 100, *Analysis of Information Elements Used in the Assessment of Certain Products of Modern Biotechnology* (1995)

No. 101, *Risk Reduction Monograph No. 2: Methylene Chloride* (1994)

No. 102, *Risk Reduction Monograph No. 3: Selected Brominated Flame Retardants* (1994)

No. 103, *Risk Reduction Monograph No. 4: Mercury* (1994)

No. 104, *Risk Reduction Monograph No. 5: Cadmium* (1994)

No. 105, *Report of the OECD Workshop on Environmental Hazard/Risk Assessment* (1995)

No. 106, *Data Requirements for Biological Pesticides* (1996)

No. 107, *Report of the OECD Workshop on the Commercialisation of Agricultural Products Derived through Modern Biotechnology* (1995)

No. 108, *Final Report on the OECD Pilot Project to Compare Pesticide Data Reviews* (1995)

No. 110, *Revised Guides for Compliance Monitoring Procedures for Good Laboratory Practice* (1995)[F, GLP]

No. 111, *Revised Guidance for the Conduct of Laboratory Inspections and Study Audits* (1995)[F, GLP]

No. 115, *Guidance for the Preparation of GLP Inspection Reports* (1995)[F, GLP]

No. 116, *The Application of the Principles of GLP to Computerised Systems* (1995)[F, GLP]

No. 117, *Industrial Products of Modern Biotechnology Intended for Release to the Environment: The Proceedings of the Fribourg Workshop* (1996)

No. 118, *Guidance Concerning Chemical Safety in Port Areas* (1996)

[Prepared in cooperation with the International Maritime Organization (IMO)]

No. 120, *Consensus Document on the Biology of Brassica Napus L (Oilseed Rape)*

No. 121, *Consensus Document on Virus Resistance through Coat Protein–mediated Protection*

OECD Priced Publications:

OECD Guidelines for Testing of Chemicals (updated 1995)^F
(OECD No. 97 93 50 1)   ISBN 92-64-14018-2   992 pages
Price in France: FF 800
Price in other countries: FF 1040   US$ 178.00   DM 300

[Also available in CD-ROM version: for more information, contact the OECD Publications Service]

Safety Evaluation of Foods Derived by Modern Biotechnology: Concepts and Principles (1993)^F
(OECD No. 93 04 1)   ISBN 92-64-13859-5   80 pages
Price in France: FF 80
Price in other countries: FF 100   US$ 19.00   DM 33

[Prepared in collaboration with the OECD Directorate for Science, Technology and Industry]

"OECD Documents" Series

Aquatic Biotechnology and Food Safety (1994)
(OECD No. 97 94 05 1)   ISBN 92-64-14063-8   100 pages
Price in France: FF 80
Price in other countries: FF 100   US$ 18.00   DM 30

[Prepared in collaboration with the OECD Directorate for Science, Technology and Industry]

Environmental Impacts of Aquatic Biotechnology (1995)
(OECD No. 97 95 14 1)   ISBN 92-64-14666-0   171 pages
Price in France: 130 FF
Price in other countries: 170 FF   US$ 35.00   DM 49   £ 22

[Prepared in collaboration with the OECD Directorate for Science, Technology and Industry.]

**Priced publications, including this OECD Document, may be ordered directly from:
OECD Publications Service, 2 rue André-Pascal, 75775 Paris Cedex 16, France.
Telex: 640 048. Telefax: (33-1) 49 10 42 76.**

In Preparation by the Environmental Health and Safety Division:

Activities to Reduce Pesticide Risks in OECD and FAO Member Countries

Guidance Document for the Conduct of Field Studies of Exposure of Pesticides in Use

Comparison of Ecological Hazard/Risk Assessment Schemes

Report of the SETAC/OECD Workshop on Avian Toxicology

The OECD Guidelines for the Testing of Chemicals (7th addendum)

Guidance Document on Dose Level Selection in Carcinogenicity Studies

Detailed Review Paper on Aquatic Toxicity Testing Methods

Report of the Final Ring Test of the Daphnia magna *Reproduction Study*

Report of the OECD Workshop on Risk Assessment and Risk Communication in the Context of Accident Prevention, Preparedness and Response

Report of the OECD/UN-ECE Workshop on Chemical Accidents

Guidance Concerning Health Aspects of Chemical Accidents

Guidance Concerning Accident Prevention, Preparation and Response at Transport Interfaces

Report of the OECD Cadmium Workshop[*]

Consensus Document on Information Used in the Assessment of Environmental Applications Involving Pseudomodas

Consensus Document on Information Used in the Assessment of Environmental Applications Involving Rhizobiacea

Consensus Document on Information Used in the Assessment of Environmental Applications Involving Bacillus

---

[*] Proposed for publication in the "OECD Documents" series.

MAIN SALES OUTLETS OF OECD PUBLICATIONS
PRINCIPAUX POINTS DE VENTE DES PUBLICATIONS DE L'OCDE

ARGENTINA – ARGENTINE
Carlos Hirsch S.R.L.
Galería Güemes, Florida 165, 4° Piso
1333 Buenos Aires Tel. (1) 331.1787 y 331.2391
Telefax: (1) 331.1787

AUSTRALIA – AUSTRALIE
D.A. Information Services
648 Whitehorse Road, P.O.B 163
Mitcham, Victoria 3132 Tel. (03) 9210.7777
Telefax: (03) 9210.7788

AUSTRIA – AUTRICHE
Gerold & Co.
Graben 31
Wien I Tel. (0222) 533.50.14
Telefax: (0222) 512.47.31.29

BELGIUM – BELGIQUE
Jean De Lannoy
Avenue du Roi 202 Koningslaan
B-1060 Bruxelles Tel. (02) 538.51.69/538.08.41
Telefax: (02) 538.08.41

CANADA
Renouf Publishing Company Ltd.
1294 Algoma Road
Ottawa, ON K1B 3W8 Tel. (613) 741.4333
Telefax: (613) 741.5439
Stores:
61 Sparks Street
Ottawa, ON K1P 5R1 Tel. (613) 238.8985
12 Adelaide Street West
Toronto, ON M5H 1L6 Tel. (416) 363.3171
Telefax: (416)363.59.63

Les Éditions La Liberté Inc.
3020 Chemin Sainte-Foy
Sainte-Foy, PQ G1X 3V6 Tel. (418) 658.3763
Telefax: (418) 658.3763

Federal Publications Inc.
165 University Avenue, Suite 701
Toronto, ON M5H 3B8 Tel. (416) 860.1611
Telefax: (416) 860.1608

Les Publications Fédérales
1185 Université
Montréal, QC H3B 3A7 Tel. (514) 954.1633
Telefax: (514) 954.1635

CHINA – CHINE
China National Publications Import
Export Corporation (CNPIEC)
16 Gongti E. Road, Chaoyang District
P.O. Box 88 or 50
Beijing 100704 PR Tel. (01) 506.6688
Telefax: (01) 506.3101

CHINESE TAIPEI – TAIPEI CHINOIS
Good Faith Worldwide Int'l. Co. Ltd.
9th Floor, No. 118, Sec. 2
Chung Hsiao E. Road
Taipei Tel. (02) 391.7396/391.7397
Telefax: (02) 394.9176

CZECH REPUBLIC – RÉPUBLIQUE TCHÈQUE
Artia Pegas Press Ltd.
Narodni Trida 25
POB 825
111 21 Praha 1 Tel. (2) 242 246 04
Telefax: (2) 242 278 72

DENMARK – DANEMARK
Munksgaard Book and Subscription Service
35, Nørre Søgade, P.O. Box 2148
DK-1016 København K Tel. (33) 12.85.70
Telefax: (33) 12.93.87

EGYPT – ÉGYPTE
Middle East Observer
41 Sherif Street
Cairo Tel. 392.6919
Telefax: 360-6804

FINLAND – FINLANDE
Akateeminen Kirjakauppa
Keskuskatu 1, P.O. Box 128
00100 Helsinki
Subscription Services/Agence d'abonnements :
P.O. Box 23
00371 Helsinki Tel. (358 0) 121 4416
Telefax: (358 0) 121.4450

FRANCE
OECD/OCDE
Mail Orders/Commandes par correspondance :
2, rue André-Pascal
75775 Paris Cedex 16 Tel. (33-1) 45.24.82.00
Telefax: (33-1) 49.10.42.76
Telex: 640048 OCDE
Internet: Compte.PUBSINQ @ oecd.org
Orders via Minitel, France only/
Commandes par Minitel, France exclusivement :
36 15 OCDE

OECD Bookshop/Librairie de l'OCDE :
33, rue Octave-Feuillet
75016 Paris Tel. (33-1) 45.24.81.81
(33-1) 45.24.81.67

Dawson
B.P. 40
91121 Palaiseau Cedex Tel. 69.10.47.00
Telefax: 64.54.83.26

Documentation Française
29, quai Voltaire
75007 Paris Tel. 40.15.70.00

Economica
49, rue Héricart
75015 Paris Tel. 45.78.12.92
Telefax: 40.58.15.70

Gibert Jeune (Droit-Économie)
6, place Saint-Michel
75006 Paris Tel. 43.25.91.19

Librairie du Commerce International
10, avenue d'Iéna
75016 Paris Tel. 40.73.34.60

Librairie Dunod
Université Paris-Dauphine
Place du Maréchal-de-Lattre-de-Tassigny
75016 Paris Tel. 44.05.40.13

Librairie Lavoisier
11, rue Lavoisier
75008 Paris Tel. 42.65.39.95

Librairie des Sciences Politiques
30, rue Saint-Guillaume
75007 Paris Tel. 45.48.36.02

P.U.F.
49, boulevard Saint-Michel
75005 Paris Tel. 43.25.83.40

Librairie de l'Université
12a, rue Nazareth
13100 Aix-en-Provence Tel. (16) 42.26.18.08

Documentation Française
165, rue Garibaldi
69003 Lyon Tel. (16) 78.63.32.23

Librairie Decitre
29, place Bellecour
69002 Lyon Tel. (16) 72.40.54.54

Librairie Sauramps
Le Triangle
34967 Montpellier Cedex 2 Tel. (16) 67.58.85.15
Telefax: (16) 67.58.27.36

A la Sorbonne Actual
23, rue de l'Hôtel-des-Postes
06000 Nice Tel. (16) 93.13.77.75
Telefax: (16) 93.80.75.69

GERMANY – ALLEMAGNE
OECD Publications and Information Centre
August-Bebel-Allee 6
D-53175 Bonn Tel. (0228) 959.120
Telefax: (0228) 959.12.17

GREECE – GRÈCE
Librairie Kauffmann
Mavrokordatou 9
106 78 Athens Tel. (01) 32.55.321
Telefax: (01) 32.30.320

HONG-KONG
Swindon Book Co. Ltd.
Astoria Bldg. 3F
34 Ashley Road, Tsimshatsui
Kowloon, Hong Kong Tel. 2376.2062
Telefax: 2376.0685

HUNGARY – HONGRIE
Euro Info Service
Margitsziget, Európa Ház
1138 Budapest Tel. (1) 111.62.16
Telefax: (1) 111.60.61

ICELAND – ISLANDE
Mál Mog Menning
Laugavegi 18, Pósthólf 392
121 Reykjavik Tel. (1) 552.4240
Telefax: (1) 562.3523

INDIA – INDE
Oxford Book and Stationery Co.
Scindia House
New Delhi 110001 Tel. (11) 331.5896/5308
Telefax: (11) 332.5993
17 Park Street
Calcutta 700016 Tel. 240832

INDONESIA – INDONÉSIE
Pdii-Lipi
P.O. Box 4298
Jakarta 12042 Tel. (21) 573.34.67
Telefax: (21) 573.34.67

IRELAND – IRLANDE
Government Supplies Agency
Publications Section
4/5 Harcourt Road
Dublin 2 Tel. 661.31.11
Telefax: 475.27.60

ISRAEL – ISRAËL
Praedicta
5 Shatner Street
P.O. Box 34030
Jerusalem 91430 Tel. (2) 52.84.90/1/2
Telefax: (2) 52.84.93

R.O.Y. International
P.O. Box 13056
Tel Aviv 61130 Tel. (3) 546 1423
Telefax: (3) 546 1442

Palestinian Authority/Middle East:
INDEX Information Services
P.O.B. 19502
Jerusalem Tel. (2) 27.12.19
Telefax: (2) 27.16.34

ITALY – ITALIE
Libreria Commissionaria Sansoni
Via Duca di Calabria 1/1
50125 Firenze Tel. (055) 64.54.15
Telefax: (055) 64.12.57
Via Bartolini 29
20155 Milano Tel. (02) 36.50.83

Editrice e Libreria Herder
Piazza Montecitorio 120
00186 Roma   Tel. 679.46.28
                          Telefax: 678.47.51

Libreria Hoepli
Via Hoepli 5
20121 Milano   Tel. (02) 86.54.46
                          Telefax: (02) 805.28.86

Libreria Scientifica
Dott. Lucio de Biasio 'Aeiou'
Via Coronelli, 6
20146 Milano   Tel. (02) 48.95.45.52
                          Telefax: (02) 48.95.45.48

JAPAN – JAPON
OECD Publications and Information Centre
Landic Akasaka Building
2-3-4 Akasaka, Minato-ku
Tokyo 107   Tel. (81.3) 3586.2016
                          Telefax: (81.3) 3584.7929

KOREA – CORÉE
Kyobo Book Centre Co. Ltd.
P.O. Box 1658, Kwang Hwa Moon
Seoul   Tel. 730.78.91
                          Telefax: 735.00.30

MALAYSIA – MALAISIE
University of Malaya Bookshop
University of Malaya
P.O. Box 1127, Jalan Pantai Baru
59700 Kuala Lumpur
Malaysia   Tel. 756.5000/756.5425
                          Telefax: 756.3246

MEXICO – MEXIQUE
OECD Publications and Information Centre
Edificio INFOTEC
Av. San Fernando no. 37
Col. Toriello Guerra
Tlalpan C.P. 14050
Mexico D.F.
            Tel. (525) 606 00 11 Extension 100
            Fax: (525) 606 13 07

Revistas y Periodicos Internacionales S.A. de C.V.
Florencia 57 - 1004
Mexico, D.F. 06600   Tel. 207.81.00
                          Telefax: 208.39.79

NETHERLANDS – PAYS-BAS
SDU Uitgeverij Plantijnstraat
Externe Fondsen
Postbus 20014
2500 EA's-Gravenhage   Tel. (070) 37.89.880
Voor bestellingen: Telefax: (070) 34.75.778

NEW ZEALAND – NOUVELLE-ZÉLANDE
GPLegislation Services
P.O. Box 12418
Thorndon, Wellington   Tel. (04) 496.5655
                          Telefax: (04) 496.5698

NORWAY – NORVÈGE
NIC INFO A/S
Bertrand Narvesens vei 2
P.O. Box 6512 Etterstad
0606 Oslo 6   Tel. (022) 57.33.00
                          Telefax: (022) 68.19.01

PAKISTAN
Mirza Book Agency
65 Shahrah Quaid-E-Azam
Lahore 54000   Tel. (42) 353.601
                          Telefax: (42) 231.730

PHILIPPINE – PHILIPPINES
International Booksource Center Inc.
Rm 179/920 Cityland 10 Condo Tower 2
HV dela Costa Ext cor Valero St.
Makati Metro Manila   Tel. (632) 817 9676
                          Telefax: (632) 817 1741

POLAND – POLOGNE
Ars Polona
00-950 Warszawa
Krakowskie Przedmieácie 7   Tel. (22) 264760
                            Telefax: (22) 268673

PORTUGAL
Livraria Portugal
Rua do Carmo 70-74
Apart. 2681
1200 Lisboa   Tel. (01) 347.49.82/5
                          Telefax: (01) 347.02.64

SINGAPORE – SINGAPOUR
Gower Asia Pacific Pte Ltd.
Golden Wheel Building
41, Kallang Pudding Road, No. 04-03
Singapore 1334   Tel. 741.5166
                          Telefax: 742.9356

SPAIN – ESPAGNE
Mundi-Prensa Libros S.A.
Castelló 37, Apartado 1223
Madrid 28001   Tel. (91) 431.33.99
                          Telefax: (91) 575.39.98

Mundi-Prensa Barcelona
Consell de Cent No. 391
08009 – Barcelona   Tel. (93) 488.34.92
                          Telefax: (93) 487.76.59

Llibreria de la Generalitat
Palau Moja
Rambla dels Estudis, 118
08002 – Barcelona
       (Subscripcions) Tel. (93) 318.80.12
       (Publicacions) Tel. (93) 302.67.23
                       Telefax: (93) 412.18.54

SRI LANKA
Centre for Policy Research
c/o Colombo Agencies Ltd.
No. 300-304, Galle Road
Colombo 3   Tel. (1) 574240, 573551-2
                   Telefax: (1) 575394, 510711

SWEDEN – SUÈDE
CE Fritzes AB
S–106 47 Stockholm   Tel. (08) 690.90.90
                          Telefax: (08) 20.50.21

Subscription Agency/Agence d'abonnements :
Wennergren-Williams Info AB
P.O. Box 1305
171 25 Solna   Tel. (08) 705.97.50
                          Telefax: (08) 27.00.71

SWITZERLAND – SUISSE
Maditec S.A. (Books and Periodicals - Livres et périodiques)
Chemin des Palettes 4
Case postale 266
1020 Renens VD 1   Tel. (021) 635.08.65
                          Telefax: (021) 635.07.80

Librairie Payot S.A.
4, place Pépinet
CP 3212
1002 Lausanne   Tel. (021) 320.25.11
                          Telefax: (021) 320.25.14

Librairie Unilivres
6, rue de Candolle
1205 Genève   Tel. (022) 320.26.23
                          Telefax: (022) 329.73.18

Subscription Agency/Agence d'abonnements :
Dynapresse Marketing S.A.
38, avenue Vibert
1227 Carouge   Tel. (022) 308.07.89
                          Telefax: (022) 308.07.99

See also – Voir aussi :
OECD Publications and Information Centre
August-Bebel-Allee 6
D-53175 Bonn (Germany)   Tel. (0228) 959.120
                          Telefax: (0228) 959.12.17

THAILAND – THAÏLANDE
Suksit Siam Co. Ltd.
113, 115 Fuang Nakhon Rd.
Opp. Wat Rajbopith
Bangkok 10200   Tel. (662) 225.9531/2
                          Telefax: (662) 222.5188

TUNISIA – TUNISIE
Grande Librairie Spécialisée
Fendri Ali
Avenue Haffouz Imm El-Intilaka
Bloc B 1 Sfax 3000   Tel. (216-4) 296 855
                          Telefax: (216-4) 298.270

TURKEY – TURQUIE
Kültür Yayinlari Is-Türk Ltd. Sti.
Atatürk Bulvari No. 191/Kat 13
Kavaklidere/Ankara
                   Tel. (312) 428.11.40 Ext. 2458
                   Telefax: (312) 417 24 90
Dolmabahce Cad. No. 29
Besiktas/Istanbul   Tel. (212) 260 7188

UNITED KINGDOM – ROYAUME-UNI
HMSO
Gen. enquiries   Tel. (171) 873 8242
Postal orders only:
P.O. Box 276, London SW8 5DT
Personal Callers HMSO Bookshop
49 High Holborn, London WC1V 6HB
                          Telefax: (171) 873 8416
Branches at: Belfast, Birmingham, Bristol,
Edinburgh, Manchester

UNITED STATES – ÉTATS-UNIS
OECD Publications and Information Center
2001 L Street N.W., Suite 650
Washington, D.C. 20036-4922 Tel. (202) 785.6323
                            Telefax: (202) 785.0350

Subscriptions to OECD periodicals may also be placed through main subscription agencies.

Les abonnements aux publications périodiques de l'OCDE peuvent être souscrits auprès des principales agences d'abonnement.

Orders and inquiries from countries where Distributors have not yet been appointed should be sent to: OECD Publications Service, 2, rue André-Pascal, 75775 Paris Cedex 16, France.

Les commandes provenant de pays où l'OCDE n'a pas encore désigné de distributeur peuvent être adressées à : OCDE, Service des Publications, 2, rue André-Pascal, 75775 Paris Cedex 16, France.

1-1996

OECD PUBLICATIONS, 2, rue André-Pascal, 75775 PARIS CEDEX 16
PRINTED IN FRANCE
(97 96 09 1) ISBN 92-64-14867-1 – No. 48733 1996